'Like all the ancient Daoist traditions, the art of classical Chinese medicine is one rooted in experiential learning. In *Heavenly Streams*, Damo Mitchell shares an inner method to access our meridians and points. It is a valuable guidebook for those interested in practicing with the subtle energies of their own bodies.'

— Master Zhongxian Wu, lifelong Daoist practitioner and author of
books on Daoist traditions, including Vital Breath of the Dao *and*
Heavenly Stems and Earthly Branches *— TianGan DiZhi*

'*Heavenly Streams* not only provides a truly comprehensive introduction to Nei Gong and Chinese medicine from the point of view of Daoism but offers the reader an effective way to understand this information within themselves.'

— Nick Lowe, practitioner of Chinese Medicine and Daoist Qi Gong instructor

'Delivered with an informal familiarity that has already sparked so many imaginations at Damo's course lectures across Europe and the United States, *Heavenly Streams* peels away Daoism's persistently obscure mystical dogma to put today's practitioners in touch with internal arts and the energetic realm.'

— Steve Galloway, Taiji teacher and owner of the Taiji Online website

T0301191

by the same author

Daoist Nei Gong
The Philosophical Art of Change
Damo Mitchell
Foreword by Dr Cindy Engel
ISBN 978 1 84819 065 8
eISBN 978 0 85701 033 9

of related interest

Fire Dragon Meridian Qigong
Essential NeiGong for Health and Spiritual Transformation
Master Zhongxian Wu and Dr Karin Taylor Wu
ISBN 978 1 84819 103 7
eISBN 978 0 85701 085 8

Chinese Shamanic Cosmic Orbit Qigong
Esoteric Talismans, Mantras, and Mudras in Healing and Inner Cultivation
Master Zhongxian Wu
ISBN 978 1 84819 056 6
eISBN 978 0 85701 059 9

Vital Breath of the Dao
Chinese Shamanic Tiger Qigong – Laohu Gong
Master Zhongxian Wu
Foreword by Chungliang Al Huang
ISBN 978 1 84819 000 9
eISBN 978 0 8570 110 7

Warrior Guards the Mountain
The Internal Martial Traditions of China, Japan and South East Asia
Alex Kozma
ISBN 978 1 84819 124 2
eISBN 978 0 85701 101 5

Heavenly
Streams

MERIDIAN THEORY IN NEI GONG

DAMO MITCHELL
Foreword by Rob Aspell

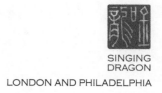

SINGING
DRAGON
LONDON AND PHILADELPHIA

First published in 2013
by Singing Dragon
an imprint of Jessica Kingsley Publishers
116 Pentonville Road
London N1 9JB, UK
and
400 Market Street, Suite 400
Philadelphia, PA 19106, USA

www.singingdragon.com

Library of Congress Cataloging in Publication Data
A CIP catalog record for this book is available from the Library of Congress

British Library Cataloguing in Publication Data
A CIP catalogue record for this book is available from the British Library

ISBN 978 1 84819 116 7
eISBN 978 0 85701 092 6

Printed and bound in Great Britain

CONTENTS

LIST OF FIGURES, TABLES AND BOXES

Figures

Tables

Boxes

FOREWORD

'Man imitates the laws of Earth, Earth imitates the laws of Heaven,
Heaven imitates the laws of Dao, Dao imitates the laws of nature (Zi Ran).'

Laozi, *Dao De Jing*, Chapter 25

Before the arrival of modern medicine, there were many traditional healing systems throughout the world that people depended on in order to treat disease. Almost all civilisations had their own methods of self-healing, and many contained similar elements in relation to developing the body's energetic system. One traditional system, which has lasted over the millennia, is that of the ancient Chinese – and the art of Daoism. Rather than solely centring their efforts on how to treat disease, the Daoists focused on preserving health and promoting longevity. It was clear to them that good health was far easier to maintain than it was to restore. Through practice and experience, they found that this should be done through self-development, cultivation of the mind and spiritual awareness. The Daoists understood that we are as one with the nature that surrounds us – a microcosm within a macrocosm. They would therefore study the laws of nature, and understand in nature the relationship between the various manifestations of Yin, Yang and the Wu Xing, and observe too how this same relationship occurs within ourselves. To me, this is reflected in Laozi's quote above. Towards the end of my Chinese medicine degree, I started to realise the extent to which modern teachings of Chinese medicine were lacking in these vital aspects. I began searching for further elaboration on the fundamental theories of Chinese medicine, but often came to a dead end, or struggled to determine the larger meaning within the classic texts. It was through Damo Mitchell that I found much of what I was looking for in the way of a deeper understanding.

I first met Damo while in the final year of my Chinese medicine degree. It was his vast knowledge of the finer details that first caught my attention. We soon struck up a friendship, with classical Chinese thought always at the heart of our conversations. My knowledge of Chinese medicine was still fresh – I was still learning. Damo seemed to have truly internalised what he knew about the Daoist arts, and was still eager to go deeper. I quickly realised that he hadn't just learnt about

Chinese medicine and Daoist philosophy, he had experienced it, and he lived it.

I had only known Damo for a short time when he kindly invited me to accompany him on a visit to China – I jumped at the opportunity. For me it was life changing. It shaped my future, and provided me with a whole new dimension to what I'd previously learnt. I would say that we grew close over that month, and I got to know Damo for who he truly is. There aren't many people of his age, or any age for that matter, with such genuine ability and understanding.

In *Heavenly Streams*, Damo continues his exploration into self-cultivation, and shares openly his understandings of the human energy system from both a Chinese medicine and a Daoist perspective. Many of the more spiritual and esoteric aspects of Chinese medicine have unfortunately been left out of institutional teachings over the years. Perhaps this is due to their more complex nature and the commitment needed to comprehend them, though ultimately they are at the heart and soul of classical Chinese thought. Damo's own commitment to the internal arts is inspiring, and thanks to his understanding through *experiential* learning, Damo distils simple thoughts from complex thoughts developed over centuries. He delivers to us his knowledge of the Daoist self-cultivation that was once a major part of what we know of as Chinese medicine. *Heavenly Streams* expands on the fundamental theories of Chinese medicine, and is welcome in bridging the gap between today's teachings and the more spiritual and esoteric practices of classical Chinese thought that are so often hard to come by, providing you with the essence of what should be followed for personal basic (and more advanced) practices.

Damo's explanations and insights are indispensible. Whether you are just beginning your journey of personal development with an interest in philosophical and spiritual thought, or even if you are a fully qualified practitioner of Chinese medicine, *Heavenly Streams* will certainly enrich your practice. I wanted to take this opportunity to thank Damo, and to say that I feel honoured to have been asked to write this Foreword. Damo deepened my understanding of Chinese medicine, and took my knowledge, and enthusiasm for that matter, to a whole new level. He has spared no effort in putting his thoughts into this book, giving many readers, who may not have had the opportunity to train with him themselves, the same in-depth and elaborate knowledge that I have had the privilege to gain in person.

Rob Aspell
Practitioner of Chinese Medicine and the Daoist Arts

ACKNOWLEDGEMENTS

First and foremost I give my eternal gratitude to all of those who have ever taught me, been taught by me or shared my journey in any way; may the continuing journey of Dao be ever smooth and flowing. Thank you to the various students who have contributed to the writing and production of this book. Thank you to Tom Burrows for being our point location model. A big thanks to Roni Edlund for helping to read the drafts and making editorial suggestions. Thank you to Ferne Brewster for tirelessly working on accurate point location diagrams and to Joe Andrews for his excellent line drawings once again. Thank you to Rob Aspell for writing the Foreword, I just hope I can live up to the kind words. Thank you to all of my students who continue to put up with my rambling teachings and lastly, much gratitude as always to Jessica Kingsley and all of the staff at Singing Dragon for having enough faith in my writing to publish this book.

DISCLAIMER

The author and publisher of this material are not responsible in any way whatsoever for any injury that may occur through reading or practising the exercises outlined in this book.

The exercises and practices may be too strenuous or risky for some people and so you should consult a qualified doctor before attempting anything from this book. It is also advised that you proceed under the guidance of an experienced teacher of the internal arts to avoid injury and confusion.

Note that any form of internal exercise is not a replacement for conventional health practices, medicines or any form of psychotherapy.

PREFACE

As I sit here typing, it is ten o'clock at night in Northern Thailand. I have just finished a few hours of intense internal arts training on the rooftops overlooking a typical Thai town. A combination of the taxing nature of the exercise I have been practising combined with the sweltering temperature has left me soaked in sweat. Pulsing waves of energy move from my centre out towards my extremities alongside waves of internal Heat which are flowing along the various channels of my meridian system. Through the years of internal training I have become as aware of my energy body as my physical body and neither one of the two is any more tangible than the other any more. In order to clear the energetic Heat from my body I bring my mind into a point near the outside of my elbows. With a gentle focus and a controlled breathing exercise I begin to feel the meridian point reacting to my mental efforts. The point begins to buzz as it activates and then the length of the meridian which the point sits upon begins to warm up. It is relieving to feel the pulsing waves within me begin to subside and the waves of internal Heat begin to lessen as my internal environment returns to a healthier state of balance. With my body temperature dropping to normal I no longer find the Thai climate so uncomfortable and so now I can sit down and write the Preface for this book, *Heavenly Streams*.

After writing my previous book, *Daoist Nei Gong: The Philosophical Art of Change*, I was both pleased and surprised at the positive response that I received. People from all over the world have begun to integrate the principles and practices outlined in the book into their daily practice. In many cases people have been surprised at the speed at which they achieved clear results once they began to study Sung breathing and other aspects of internal work from the system I teach. Some of these people have travelled to attend training events with me and have begun to move even deeper into Daoist internal practices such as the meditative art of alchemy.

When wondering how to follow up *Daoist Nei Gong* with a second book on the internal arts I decided to once again focus on some of the pieces of information which are not currently so easy to access in the Western world. Originally I was going to begin writing about the meditative practices of Daoism but then it struck me that it would be far more useful to focus on one small yet important aspect of Nei Gong and Qi Gong which is often left out of many people's practice; this is the practice of connecting with, feeling and adjusting the energy body directly using the consciousness. This practice sits somewhere between Qi Gong, meditation and the lesser known art of Shen Gong. A great many of the emails I received after the last book I wrote were from people wondering how they were going to progress deeper into their practice when they could not feel their own Qi. Some of these messages even stressed that they had thought of the meridian system as a purely conceptual framework rather than a literal part of the human body system which could be felt and worked with. In response to these concerns I present to you here *Heavenly Streams*, a book which contains step-by-step instructions on how to experience the benefits of working directly with the various elements which make up your energy body.

As with all practices, results take time. The exercises contained within this book should be considered moderate to advanced in difficulty level. Ten minutes will yield very few results but yet those who commit the time and their focus to these practices will soon find that they have given themselves a direct way to access and change their internal environment on a very deep level.

I hope that this book can be of some benefit to the internal arts community in general, whether that be practitioners of Qi Gong, Nei Gong, Taijiquan or Chinese medicine. I have had to include a fair amount of information which crosses into all four of these areas of the Daoist tradition. Where possible I have attempted to keep information only to that which is absolutely essential. Practitioners of traditional Chinese medicine should also note that some of the information contained within this book differs a little from that which they may have been taught. This is to be expected from such an ancient tradition which developed over so many centuries across such a large geographical area. Different teachers emphasise different principles. Where applicable I have made clear where information within this book differs from the common understanding.

I am primarily a practitioner of the Daoist arts rather than a theorist and I am certainly no writer! Consequently I apologise in advance for the lack of eloquence in my writing style and for any areas of the book which are confusing or unclear.

Happy practice.

Chiang Mai, Thailand

INTRODUCTION TO THE HEAVENLY STREAMS

This is not an instructional book on Chinese medicine, neither is it a book purely on the subject of Qi Gong. Rather, it is a guide to the traditional methods of study which underpinned both of these practices within the ancient Daoist lineages; lineages which, unbroken for centuries, transmitted a complex catalogue of the human energetic system.

It is a great boon within modern times that we have access to all kinds of information. At the touch of a button we can read about absolutely anything without leaving our own homes. Information which would previously have been either out of our reach or would have required years of dedicated searching is now ours to have within the space of a few seconds. Within the world of the internal arts this means that anybody can have all of the available information in front of them when they begin their studies. In the past, masters of the ancient traditions selected their students carefully and teachings were preserved through close, one to one tuition. It would have been impossible for a casual student of Qi Gong to learn the theory and practices of Daoism without first seeking out a true master and convincing them to take them on as an apprentice.

The positive side of this is that anybody can gain the benefits of these wonderful arts. People all over the world can experience the profound beauty of practices once confined to the mountains of China; the health benefits of Qi Gong, Nei Gong, Taijiquan and more have spread to the corners of the globe. To balance this out there are several negatives. For every Yang there must be a Yin. First, people have access to information too early; many contemporary students of the internal arts do not spend enough time building a foundation in the basics as they are in too much of a hurry to reach the higher levels that they may openly read about. The more mundane stages of working with the physical body and the breath are skimmed over as they begin to try and work directly with the energy body and consciousness. Second and most important, experiential understanding is often replaced with mere intellectual knowledge. Too many people read about an area of Daoism and then presume that they have fully understood the concept. This book is an attempt at an answer to this weakness in the modern way of learning the internal arts.

A major part of the foundational knowledge for Qi Gong or Nei Gong is having an understanding of the energy body and in particular the meridian system. Anybody familiar with any form of Chinese medicine will already be comfortable with the concept of the meridians and most likely have an in depth knowledge of their pathways and the location of the various points which sit along these meridians. It is most likely that this knowledge is gained from spending great amounts of time studying various charts and diagrams. This knowledge is then transferred onto the human body during the course of their work giving them a working understanding of the effects of different points when they are stimulated on their patients. What is less likely is that they studied the meridian system through an experiential exploration of the meridians using focused self-awareness. Understanding the energy body should be of prime importance to students of any of the internal arts and internal exploration should be a major part of the process of attaining this knowledge. In these times when all of the collective theories of the energy body can be had very quickly, true experiential understanding has sadly become quite rare.

In order to understand the energy body we must first understand the way in which it is formed. We need to explore the spiritual energies of the five elements. Far more than just a conceptual framework these five vibrational patterns form the blueprints for the complex network of energetic pathways which connect our mind and body to the wider cosmos within which we live. Within this book I explore the nature of the five elements, the meridians and the meridian points of the body while inviting the reader to experience their nature through guided internal exercises using the body, breath and mind.

Although much of the information within this book sits somewhere between Nei Gong and Chinese medicine I have attempted to restrict the information to only that which is necessary. I did not wish to shut out those who had no knowledge of Chinese medical theory and so I have kept in only the knowledge which is required to understand the energy body and the nature of imbalance within its various pathways.

It is a sad fact that many people are living in a state of perpetual ill health. In the Western world conditions which often originate from poor emotional states and poor lifestyles evolve into more serious conditions. Those living in these states are usually forced to rely on either Western medicine or alternative therapists to treat these conditions. Completely disempowered by a lack of connection to their own body, those with poor health are too often consuming various forms of medication or going for regular hands on treatments seeking temporary pain relief. If, however, we are able to connect to and transform the nature of our own energy body through practised internal exercises then we are often able to cut off imbalance before it develops into more serious illness. The empowering act of contacting and exploring your own energy body can not only show you the nature of your own Qi but also give you a way to change and rebalance it. Qi Gong is one such method of doing this but it requires that we have attained the stage of feeling and moving our own energy using the power of our mind; the practice of working directly with the Heavenly Streams.

BOX 1.1: WHO SHOULD NOT TRAIN

While the practices in this book can be of great benefit to the majority of people, there are still some who should not carry out these exercises. The internal arts can, in some cases, carry risks and so the following people should not practise the methods I have outlined here.

I am not a great fan of children or teenagers practising any more than the absolute basics of Qi Gong. The practices within this book should really be considered intermediate to advanced in difficulty and so please do not practise these methods if you are under 18 years of age. Within my own school I never take any students under this age for anything other than external practices. The teenage years in particular are a period of emotional development. A young person's consciousness is in such a state of flux that deep internal work during this stage of development runs the risk of disturbing their natural emotional development. Having seen and experienced some of the dangers here myself I am cautious not to go beyond the basics of the Daoist arts with children and teenagers.

I cannot make clear enough my views on pregnant women practising the Daoist internal arts. I am absolutely against it. I immediately stop any of my female students who become pregnant from training in deep internal work with me. They are only allowed to stretch and work on the physical side of the arts. A practice such as Yoga would be far more beneficial while pregnant. While it is quite possible that there would be no problem for a pregnant woman to practise Qi Gong or Nei Gong I cannot guarantee it. There is a great deal of energetic change going on for a woman at this time and the Qi of the abdomen is very fragile. I do not feel that it is worth taking any risks at this time with internal practices. You may note that in the lists of meridian points contained within this book some are contra-indicated during pregnancy. I have included these as they are classical contra-indications but in fact I would consider direct access of any of the points using the Yi contra-indicated during pregnancy.

Those with a history of mental illness should be careful when beginning any internal work and seek guidance from an experienced teacher throughout. Any form of work with the mind can be damaging to those with a mental illness if it is not carried out correctly.

You should also not train when sick or when in an emotionally heightened state. Wait until your illness is passed or you have reached a more stable emotional state prior to beginning practice.

CHAPTER 1

THE DAO OF
UNDERSTANDING

It is in the nature of human beings to explore their own inner environment. This can clearly be seen when looking back at any of the ancient cultures that have flourished throughout history. The study of spirituality and the nature of consciousness has manifested in countless different ways and systems which were traditionally passed down from teacher to student. In this way the ancient teachings were preserved as each generation of teachers added to the collective wisdom of their ancestors with their own inspired understandings. The Daoist school of China is one such tradition which heralds from the teachings of the mythical sage, Laozi who is said to have lived in the sixth century BCE. This tradition, along with Buddhism and Confucianism, had a great impact upon Chinese culture; echoes of its teachings can still be seen permeating their society today. Many of the arts and practices which were born from Daoism have also survived to this day including such treasures as Qi Gong, Taijiquan and Chinese medicine; practices which have spread outside of China to the rest of the world.

In modern times there has been a shift in emphasis towards the study of science. The ways of spiritual development have been relegated to a place of lesser importance and, alongside them, the arts which were born from the wisdom of the ancients. In order to survive this shift in attitude many of the Daoist arts sought to adapt with the times. Adaptation along with the changing trends of society is a treasured ideal within the philosophy of the Daoists and in this way arts such as Qi Gong and Chinese medicine have survived. Partly embracing the findings of modern science, the principles and reasoning behind many of the practices differ greatly from their original tenets. While many of their benefits can still be had by modern people, the arts are but a pale shadow of what they have the potential to be.

The Dao of Understanding

There are two main ways to approach the study of the Daoist arts: from a purely intellectual approach or from an experiential approach. In modern times the emphasis is upon intellectual study. We seek to give everything a clear definition based upon conclusions reached from observation and, often, scientific study. In ancient times understanding was given more credence if it was based upon experiential knowledge.

If we apply these two different approaches to an art which was born from the Daoist school, Chinese medicine, we can see how the past and present ways of study differ.

In contemporary Chinese medicine, which is usually known as TCM, students study the various theories which underpin the practice from books and charts. Students are often taught the underlying theories such as: Yin and Yang, five elements, Zang Fu (organ) theory and so on, straight from textbooks. They are taught that these theories were developed from an observation of natural phenomena within the external environment and over years of experimentation they came up with a form of medicine that worked effectively. Meridians and the points which run along these energetic pathways are learnt from books and students usually spend time drawing these points onto each other or memorising their location according to anatomical landmarks. In this way, Chinese medicine is studied purely intellectually with much of the theory learnt 'parrot fashion'. While this purely intellectual way of studying Chinese medicine has its place, it is also extremely limiting.

The ancient approach to Chinese medicine differs greatly from the modern way of learning. Students are encouraged to first explore the nature of their own energy system prior to beginning their work on other people's. Through training their awareness to 'go inside' and get in touch with the energetic pathways which flow through their bodies students are enabled to feel the way that energy or Qi moves within them. Over time they can begin to feel how the concepts of Yin, Yang and the five elements are actual energetic states which are governed by this flow of Qi through the meridian system. Intellectual understanding comes only after experiential understanding. This way of studying Chinese medicine has no real basis in science; instead it is based upon a set of teachings which stretches far back into the mists of time. These teachings come from a tradition formed from the collective wisdom of the past masters of Daoism who did not limit their mind with definitions but rather expanded their minds with the artistic poetry born from experiential learning.

As with Chinese medicine, arts such as Qi Gong and Taijiquan also went through a similar process of adaptation to suit the needs of modern people. The same process of experiential learning was replaced with intellectual study and so their development was halted. What is presented in this book is a methodology for approaching the study of the Daoist arts from the ancient way of experiential exploration. This is the Dao of understanding.

Inner Study

The Daoist arts are widespread and diverse; they incorporate the study of the nature of everything which exists between Heaven and Earth. It would be possible to study the Daoist tradition in detail for several lifetimes and still only begin to touch upon a fragment of the different elements which make up this magnificent school of thought. Some areas of study, however, are considered universally important to all Daoist arts. Two of these are the nature of the human energetic system and the movement of the two powers of Yin and Yang.

It is an interesting characteristic of existence that life repeats itself on every level. That which takes place within the wider macrocosm of the universe is directly reflected within the microcosm of the human body. The same force which dictates and directs the movements of the stars and planets also shifts various energies within the human mind and body. This force is known as Qi and without it life in all its various forms would cease to exist. The ancient cultures of the world understood this intrinsic link between human beings and the wider environment. The Daoists were no exception and all of their many arts, practices and philosophies are based upon this rule of micro and macro systems. The ancient Daoists studied the shifting energies of the skies above them and grew to understand how all life upon Earth not only relies upon the movements of Heaven but also how it matches it on every level.

If you take a holographic image and cut it into pieces you are not left with a small part of the original image as would be the case with a photo. Instead you are left with various miniature representations of the original hologram in its entirety. No matter how small the individual pieces each will contain the entire original image. The Daoists viewed existence in the same way as one large, organic hologram of which human beings are but one, very small, part. If we view life in this way then we can understand how it is possible, through the study of any one part, to gain an understanding of the whole.

To study the shifting nature of energy as it moved throughout the entire universe would be an impossibly vast task whereas studying the nature of energy throughout the meridian system and human body is far more manageable. It is for this reason that meridian study was considered foundational knowledge for any of the Daoist arts. It was also believed that if this study was taken far enough then it would lead to a deep comprehension of the nature of the wider universe; an understanding which was said to be the basis for spiritual illumination.

The Human Energy System

Far more than just the physical body which is understood within Western scientific thought, we have a complex network of energetic pathways flowing through us. These pathways work together to carry a vibrational wave of information, Qi, to the various organs and tissues of the body along with the blood and body fluids which our physical body needs to exist. This energetic system has been studied within numerous cultures throughout history but arguably the Daoist concepts which have survived to this day offer the most complete and in depth information as to its nature.

These are the meridian pathways used within practices such as acupuncture and Shiatsu as well as within moving exercises such as Qi Gong and Taijiquan. As well as governing the health and internal balance of our body they also connect us to the external environment making us an integrated part of the wider universe. They were often seen as providing a link to the shifting energies of the Heavens and for this reason they are also known as 'Heavenly Streams'. This connection between the external environment and the energetic pathways which flow through us takes place at various points on the body; points that can be accessed with either a needle, as in the case of acupuncture, pressure, as in massage, or with the mind, as in Daoist internal exercises.

The various pathways of the meridian system were studied within the Daoist schools and then mapped out through countless hours of internal exploration. Figure 1.1 shows the human energetic system according to the Daoist tradition.

Flowing through these pathways are the various forms of energy or Qi which are directly worked with within all of the Daoist arts. Qi sits at the mid-point between human consciousness and the physical body, providing a link between these two aspects of human existence. Daoist arts work on the principle that if we are able to access and work with the Qi of our body then we will be able to draw together both mind and body into one integrated whole as shown in Figure 1.2.

Unity is the way to good health and spiritual elevation while division moves us towards our decline; this is the key ethos which underpins all Daoist arts. Qi is the key to achieving this because of its position in the centre between mind and body. It is almost impossible for the physical body to communicate directly with our consciousness without the aid of

Qi which acts as the messenger between the two. This means that working with our physical body alone will not give us direct access to the state of our consciousness while working purely on the level of consciousness will not enable us to greatly improve our physical health. If, however, we are able to access our Qi then we are able to bring about change to both physicality and our own consciousness.

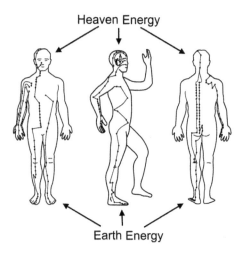

Figure 1.1: The Human Energetic System

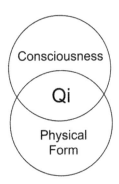

Figure 1.2: Qi, Consciousness and Physicality

The Three Treasures

These three elements of consciousness, energy and physicality are known as the three treasures within Daoist thought and known respectively as: Shen, Qi and Jing. Since everything within the microcosm of the body must be matched within the macrocosm of the external environment then there must also be three external treasures. These are known as: Heaven, Man and Earth. Figure 1.3 shows the micro and macro manifestations of the three treasures.

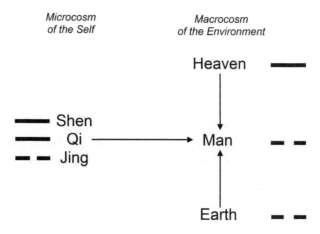

Figure 1.3: The Three Treasures

In the same way that working with our Qi enables us to bring together consciousness (Shen) and our physical body (Jing), working with the middle treasure of Man enables us to bring together the treasures of Heaven and Earth. If we can bring together these two powers then we have attained a profound level of attainment within the Daoist arts. The middle, macrocosmic treasure of Man is worked with by studying the energy system and bringing it into balance. This is the aim of Daoist arts such as Qi Gong (Energy work), Nei Gong (Internal skill) and Nei Dan Gong (Daoist meditation).

The Rubbish of Daoism

If we seek to understand the energy system then we must also seek to understand its nature when it is out of balance. Imbalances within the energy system manifest as disease, both of the mind and the body since Qi sits between these two. All sickness, according to Daoism, is anchored somewhere in the energetic body and clearing this imbalance will begin to shift the disease. Because working with the body's Qi begins to improve the health of the mind and the body, the Daoist arts became widespread within the population. Practices such as Qi Gong became popular with those who wanted to either prevent or cure sickness. It is interesting to note though that this was not the original goal of the Daoist arts; it was a by-product. Good health and longevity, for which Daoism became well known, were originally just stepping stones to further practices and in many cases were actually spoken of as the 'rubbish of Daoism'. This is not to say that attaining good health is not important, of course it is, it is just interesting to understand that within Daoism this was only the first step. A step which resulted from the 'middle treasure' of Man becoming balanced so that the powers of Heaven and Earth could be connected to.

If we understand this then it is clear to see how an understanding of the nature of disease according to Daoist thought is an integral part of all other Daoist arts regardless of whether you are interested in the medicinal arts or not. Practitioners of arts such as Qi Gong, Nei Gong or even the internal martial arts should all have knowledge of Chinese medicine if they ever wish to proceed past the early stages in their practices. A study of the nature of imbalance will ultimately lead towards moving into a state of balance. Once again this reflects the relationship of Yin and Yang.

Tuning the Mind

Reality as we experience it is dictated by the level of vibration which we are able to tune in to. Within classical Daoist thought (but not contemporary Chinese medicine) one of the functions of the brain was to serve as a sort of radio which was able to tune in to different frequencies. The functions of the brain are discussed in further detail in Chapter 7. When we begin our practice, the majority of us are tuned solely into the physical realm. Our mind is only able to pick up the denser frequencies which relate to physical matter. Our reality is dictated by that which we can see, feel or experience directly with our senses. Scientists seek to explore the nature of this reality in greater depth by creating increasingly powerful microscopes which can show us the nature of the physical world at minute levels. We have managed to zoom in so close that we have now managed to see the ultimate truth of physicality: it doesn't really exist. Over 99 per cent of each atom which makes up the physical realm is actually emptiness, it is not there. As the modern mind seeks to explore this realm in greater detail, struggling to understand the nature of reality, it has missed out one vitally important fact: physicality is only one realm of existence. The physical realm is only a fraction of the world we live in and until the mind is tuned in to the frequency of the next realm, that of energy, we are still only focusing on one small area. The energetic realm sits a step higher in the frequency range than the physical world and then the realm of pure consciousness sits higher again; beyond this lie Heaven and Dao.

BOX 1.1: PERSONAL RESPONSIBILITY

Within Daoism, the microcosm of the human body and the macrocosm of the external world are no different from each other; they are one and the same. That which manifests inside of us manifests outside of us as well. This holistic, connected view of human people and the cosmos therefore states that the more damage that we do to our environment, the sicker we become and vice versa.

Environmental disasters both natural and man-made are constantly a feature within our news. Natural resources are running low and numerous species of animals have become extinct due to excessive hunting, pollution or destruction of natural habitats like the rainforest. The Daoist view is that this damage to the outside world has to be reflected back onto human beings. It is true that we are living in a time where being 'healthy' is actually quite rare. Vast numbers of people in the Western world are reliant on all sorts of medication and the rate of obesity is rapidly increasing along with various life-threatening diseases. Is there a connection here? The Daoist view of microcosmic to macrocosmic connection says that there has to be. The energy which flows through both us and our world ensures that the information outside also flows within. In the same way, a natural disregard for our own health will begin to have a knock on effect to the planet we live within.

The responsibility therefore falls to each and every person, according to Daoist thought, as taking care of our own health also helps the energy of the world we live within. When people lose respect for themselves they also lose respect for the world we live within which is a terrible shame as it is a truly beautiful place.

The responsibility for personal health also has meaning when we look at the nature of Jing. According to Daoist thought, congenital essence is in part passed on to you by your parents. If your essence is weak then it is likely that your children will also have weak essence and so poor health, a low immune system and a shorter natural lifespan. Essence also goes deeper than this as it also has a kind of memory; it stores information. This information is said to be passed on to the next generation or even the generation after this. The result is that your actions can have a direct effect upon your children and your grandchildren. Perhaps you are one of those people who thinks they are very lucky as they are able to eat as much as they like without gaining any weight? According to Daoist thought this would make the chances of your children and grandchildren having digestive or weight disorders very likely as the information stored within the essence was passed to them. In the same way, somebody who could smoke cigarettes for years without having any lung complaints would likely cause the generations after them to have seriously deficient Lung Qi. Countless negative actions such as this can be passed on through the information stored within the essence. The responsibility for both the health of the planet and of future generations sits with all of us.

It is interesting that children are born with a strong connection to the energetic realm. Their mind enables them to feel and connect with higher frequency vibrations. They naturally tend to be more intuitive as they read the energy systems of people they meet. Like children, animals are more connected than adult humans and are easily able to read the shifting energies of the environment. As we age we are taught to use our brain in a less intuitive way. Through education and the lessons given to us by our peers and family we are trained to define everything in the limited way which prevails throughout modern culture. Gradually these learnt biases begin to adjust the way our mind perceives reality; the tuning of the mind decreases and we are only able to perceive the physical world.

One of our first steps in the Daoist arts is to re-train this side of our mind and adjust the frequency which we are able to pick up. We need to reconnect to the energetic realm and the way we do this is to first reconnect to our own energy body.

Once we are able to connect to our own energetic system then we can begin to learn to adjust the energy flowing through it. When this energy begins to change it has a knock on effect on both our consciousness and the physical body.

Re-attaining Inner Balance

As discussed above, attaining good health is the first step on the road towards union with Dao. Figure 1.4 shows the progressive stages towards union with Dao.

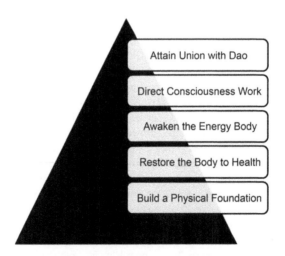

Figure 1.4: The Foundation of Health

In order to enable my students to begin working towards inner balance I teach the stages of attainment in the following sequence. Although traditionally there is no particular sequence, I have found it useful to teach in this way.

1. Prepare and Relax the Mind and Body

2. Five Element Practice

3. Connect the Yi to the Breath

4. Access the Energy Body

5. Explore the Energy Body

6. Understand Your Internal Environment

7. Begin to Adjust the Inner Environment

8. Develop

Every teacher has their own way of passing on knowledge; personally I like practices which can be laid out in steps like this. It gives structure to beginning students who can otherwise find the scope of the Daoist arts overwhelming. The series of stages is only a guideline; it is possible that some of these stages will take place in a slightly different order due to people's individual nature.

Prepare and Relax the Mind and Body

Before any practice can be carried out we must first get into the correct state. Our body must be loose, relaxed and comfortable with open and flexible joints. Our mind should be as quiet and calm as we can make it prior to the practice so that it is not distracted by outside thoughts. This is always the first step in any Daoist practice and in many ways the most difficult one.

Five Element Practice

Included in the next chapter are five exercises known as the Wu Xing Qi Gong. These five simple exercises aim to regulate the five elemental energies of the body. I have found through experience that these particular exercises taken from the medical Qi Gong school of thought are particularly useful for addressing any obvious elemental disturbances prior to beginning the more advanced practices outlined within this book.

Connect the Yi to the Breath

Our Yi is our level of mental focus and awareness. Through practice we are able to link this awareness to our breathing which can then be directed via the breath through the energy system. This gives us a tangible way to move our mind throughout the energy body in the early stages of our practice. At later stages of attainment this is no longer needed and the Yi can move independently of the breath.

Access the Energy Body

There are several points on the body which are easy access points for our awareness. Once we are able to connect our mind to these points they will help us to access the energy body; in particular the meridians. This requires a strong knowledge of the location of the points combined with a strong Yi and effective breathing techniques. If we can access the energy body via these points we will be able to move on to the stage of exploring the energy system.

Explore the Energy Body

For many this is a groundbreaking stage. Many students who I have taught to reach this stage have been practising acupuncturists, Qi Gong practitioners and so forth who have worked with their energy body for many years. Although they may have understood the meridian system very well from a theoretical perspective many of them have never actually connected with it. At this stage the entire meridian you are connecting with opens up and can be felt as easily as the physical body. Now it is possible to move your awareness along the line of the meridian and explore the different sensations at the meridian points which sit along its pathway. With practice it is possible to feel how every little change in the movement of Qi in each meridian affects the rest of the system.

Understand Your Internal Environment

Once you have explored the nature of your own energy body you are able to see the nature of your internal environment. It becomes clear to see which organs may have the strongest or weakest energy, which emotions affect you the most and which ones have taken the biggest toll on your health. You can understand how you relate to certain climates, conditions and food. From this you can understand the nature of your relationship to the powers of Heaven and Earth.

Begin to Adjust the Inner Environment

The next step is to bring about change to any imbalances you have identified in order to bring your body back to a state of harmony. This is achieved through controlled use of the mind and the breath and an understanding of the meridian points of the body. This is the link between Daoist alchemy and Chinese medicine.

Develop

Once a foundation has been built in the above stages it is time to begin moving deeper into the arts. From here it is possible to take your practice in many directions. Those interested in medicine will by now have a great experiential understanding of the nature of the energy system; this is invaluable for those who work within the field of Chinese medicine. Those interested in practices such as Qi Gong, Nei Gong or meditation will have the tools needed to move on from this state of inner balance to higher levels of practice. Developing an understanding of the energy body is a major part of comprehending the nature of your own personal microcosm. If we are able to understand the way that our own microcosm works we are able, in turn, to understand the nature of the outer universe within which we live. This is the principle upon which all Daoist internal practices are based.

CHAPTER 2

THE FIVE LIGHTS

According to Daoist thought, human beings do not exist as stand-alone entities. Our birth, existence, personal evolution and eventual demise are both dependent upon and an integral part of the ebb and flow of the energies of the universe. Human beings sit at a point between Heaven and Earth, a point of connection between the great powers of Yin and Yang. How well we understand this concept and integrate it into our life and actions will dictate not only our health and well-being but also to what extent we will evolve spiritually over the course of our lives.

This connection to the environment begins at the point of our conception. The Yin and Yang energies of our parents combine to begin the formation of a new person. Working together in harmony these two forces interact to form the various elements which will go on to form the various physical, energetic and conscious components which make up a unified being. Nourished in the fertile Yin environment of our mother's womb for nine months we gradually develop until it is time to be born into the outside world. Throughout this process of development the Yang energies of the Heavens pour down into us and begin to form into the various aspects of consciousness which will give us cognition, insight and understanding. This is a time of balance and beginning, creation and harmonisation.

After birth the intermingling of Heaven and Earth continues. The air we breathe and food we consume along with the mental stimulation, support and love we receive each day during our early years begins to develop the way in which we understand the world. The delicate balance of internal energies mapped out within the Daoist school of thought change and transform through alchemical processes to create individuality. As we grow and age we experience increasing degrees of external stimuli which continue to affect us internally throughout our lives. This is the process of living.

The Daoist view is that our role is to develop spiritually. The function of human existence is to strive for illumination. This is the natural development which needs to take place if we are ever to realise our true potential as unlimited spiritual beings. Throughout our lives we should be seeking to balance the energies which are in a state of constant flux within us and transmute them into increasingly more ethereal substances. This is the path of union and the way to Dao which has been practised throughout the ages by Daoist priests from their initial shamanic practices through to the alchemical meditative arts which form a basis for so many of China's philosophies and arts.

Understanding Heaven and Earth

Everything within the universe is viewed as an interaction between the two energies known as Yin and Yang. Yin is a force of decline and stillness, silence and all that is calm while Yang pertains to movement and creativity, action and change. Within the Daoist view of creation, Yin and Yang divided into separate entities from the original state of being, known as Wuji, which is shown in Figure 2.1.

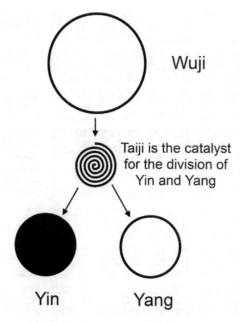

Figure 2.1: Yin, Yang and Wuji

Wuji is understood as the point at which the grand potential of Dao makes itself present within the spiritual realm. It is a point of stillness that exists above Yin and Yang and yet has no geographical location of its own. Wuji is the seed for all of the realms of existence which are born from it.

Yang was the more ethereal of the two powers and rose to form the Heavens. Yin was denser and so sank down to form the Earth. Between these two poles every possible interaction between Yin and Yang began to take place. Energy swirled and moved together. Change and development took place and thus existence was born. These intermingling energies became known as Qi to the ancient Daoists. They noted that Qi was essentially a vibrational force that motivated everything within the universe. Different vibrations could be mapped out as different combination of positives and negatives, peaks and troughs. Each of these different vibrations contained information which moved throughout everything and created life as we know it.

All of the different combinations of Yin and Yang vibrational information or 'Qi' were mapped out; first into eight broad categories and then later into 64 variations. These 64 variations became known as the Hexagrams. These are shown in Figure 2.2.

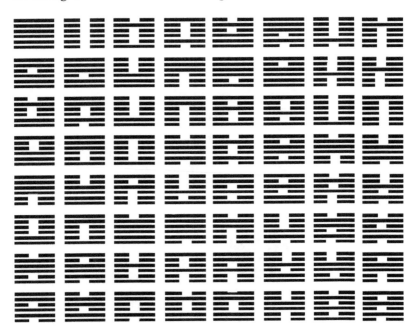

Figure 2.2: The Hexagrams

Through the study of the movement of the Hexagrams the ancient Daoists were able to reach great levels of understanding regarding the nature of Qi within the macrocosm of the universe as well as within the microcosm of the human body. They understood how health and harmony relied upon there being healthy movement and transformation of energy within the body. They came to realise how the movements of energy within the environment could empower a human being towards spiritual elevation or disable them with sickness depending upon whether or not a person understood how to live alongside the fluctuating powers of Heaven and Earth.

The energy which flows between Heaven and Earth affects us in countless ways. We are both a product of and an integral part of the wider cosmos. The lighter more ethereal energies are closer to Yang/Heaven and so have a more direct relationship with our consciousness while the denser more Yin energies are closer to Earth and so affect us on a more physical level. Everything in between relates more closely to our energy system – the network of meridians which is utilised within therapies such as acupuncture or practices such as Qi Gong.

The ideal way for a human being to relate to Heaven and Earth is for them to become a conduit for their movements and activities. A balanced human being free of tensions and blockages within their energy body will simply allow the Qi from above and below to flow through them and meet within their centre. The free-flow of Yin and Yang energies will serve to nourish the mind and body. Stagnation will be transmuted into fluidity enabling a person to move forward with their lives in the healthiest possible manner. Imbalance and blockages within the body will mean that a person is disconnected from Heaven and Earth; this is the route to ill health. This concept of becoming a conduit for Heaven and Earth is explored later in this book.

Heaven Energy

Consciousness is seen as a gift from Heaven. Chinese astrology tells us that the position of certain planets and stars at the time of our birth has a direct effect upon our nature. Not only this, but it also gives us a certain predisposition to certain elemental energies and imbalances. To the Daoists birth was accompanied by a rush of cosmic energy that descends from the Heavens and enters our consciousness body. This is the energy of Shen or 'spirit' which is the most Yang and ethereal energetic substance to form part of us. Shen within Daoist thoughts forms a comprehensive and detailed picture of the human psyche. Unlike many Western traditions which refer to any aspect of the spirit or soul in a very abstract manner, Daoism has an almost anatomical view of human consciousness. Shen has a direct effect upon every part of our being and every action we undertake. It governs our thought processes, our emotional make-up, our level of comprehension and countless other tasks generally associated with the mind within Western thought. Unlike the generally understood view of the mind within this part of the world, the Shen not only has a direct influence upon the body but aspects of it are also housed within different physical organs of the body.

Energy is constantly changing. Nothing is constant. Shen is no exception. When Shen begins to condense it lowers in vibrational frequency and becomes known as Qi. This energy then flows throughout the meridian system of the body reaching the various organs of the body and animating our physical form. Qi flows throughout our body like rivers and streams via the various energetic pathways which we will study in detail within this book. Providing this energy flows freely we will remain in a state of health and well-being. If, however, this energy becomes blocked or deficient for any reason then the flow will no longer be harmonious and smooth. Stagnation occurs and illness develops. Returning ourselves to health relies on us being able to free up our meridian system and once more restore a healthy flow of Qi.

If Qi becomes any denser it forms what we know as Jing. Jing is the densest of the three categories of energetic substance. It is the closest to physical matter and the base construct of all life. Jing can be seen as our essence, it is the fuel which keeps us going. If our Jing is allowed to run low then we once again experience sickness. Jing depletion is particularly prevalent within modern society which is stressful and does not place enough importance upon mental rest. Jing is often linked closely to the kidneys and the adrenals which are easily burnt out by excessive stress.

Earth Energy

The energy of Earth is largely given to us through the food we eat. Everything we eat contains a different type of Qi and so has different properties. It is from this understanding that food therapy was developed in ancient China and from this herbal medicine. Unlike Western nutrition which focuses upon the vitamins and minerals contained within food Daoists studied the nature of food according to its energetic properties.

The second key way in which Earth energy is drawn into the body is through our connection with the planet itself. The bases of our feet have two points known as Yongquan (KI1). These serve to draw energy directly from beneath us into the meridian system and primarily the Kidneys. This energy nourishes the body with healing energy; practices such as Taijiquan, Qi Gong and Nei Gong can help to strengthen this drawing in of Earth Qi into the body.

Figure 2.3 shows how Heaven and Earth energy comes into the body.

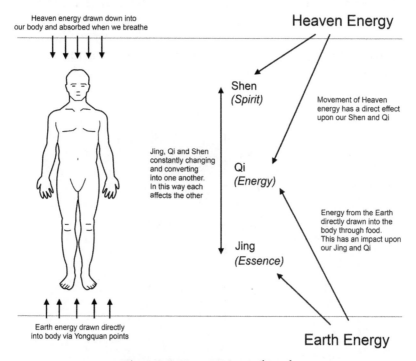

Figure 2.3: Heaven, Man and Earth

The figure shows that Jing, Qi and Shen convert into one another within the body. Essentially they are all the same thing; different vibrational frequencies of the same universal energy. As each is information, imbalance within one may affect the others. For example, an emotional disturbance which affects a person's Shen will over time begin to disrupt the flow of Qi within the body. This will have an effect within the Jing level of the body which will result in physical illness developing. The same process works the other way around. Unhealthy food or overstrain will in time effect a person's Jing reserves. This will result in blockages and imbalance within the energy system and so the Qi will be negatively affected. This will in time lead to a Shen disturbance and so the mind will become imbalanced.

Figure 2.4 shows how each of the three internal treasures of Jing, Qi and Shen are simply more or less refined versions of the same vibrational information.

If the vibration of Jing decreases further it will 'condense' to form physical matter and eventually the extreme Yin manifestation of Earth. In the same way, if the frequency of Shen is increased it will align with the energy of Heaven and, then finally, Dao itself. Understanding this enables you to see how man sits between Heaven and Earth and how we are simply a combination of the information moving between these two extremes. This view is the basis not only for the practices in this book but also for all of the Daoist arts.

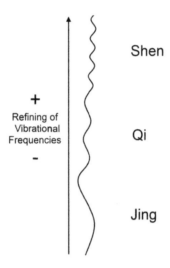

Figure 2.4: Vibrational Frequencies

The Five Spiritual Lights

According to Daoist thought conscious life originates within the realm of Dao. From here it is passed down into the great potential energy which is Wuji. Wuji sits at the threshold between Dao and the consciousness realm. The consciousness realm sits at the highest level of frequency above the energetic and finally the physical realm. This is shown in Figure 2.5.

When this gift of spiritual essence is passed from Dao into Wuji it is known as 'seed consciousness'. As it moves through Wuji into the consciousness realm it begins to divide into five different parts known within Daoism as the 'five spiritual lights'. This is the first refraction of many which take place within the process of constructing the human mind.

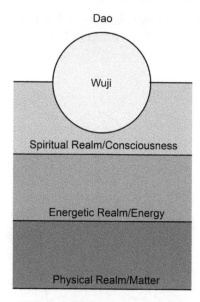

Figure 2.5: Dao, Wuji and the Three Realms

These five spiritual lights are themselves different combinations of Yin and Yang which take on individual characteristics. The five spiritual lights are named: Shen, Yi, Po, Zhi and Hun. At this level of manifestation they are five different coloured lights which have been split from the bright golden brilliance of unified consciousness which exists beyond the spiritual realm. Table 2.1 lists the colours associated with the five spiritual lights.

Table 2.1: The Five Spiritual Lights

Light	Shen	Yi	Po	Zhi	Hun
Colour	Red	Yellow	White	Blue	Green
Movement	Expanding	Dividing	Contracting	Sinking	Thrusting
Element	Fire	Earth	Metal	Water	Wood

As these lights move down into the energetic realm they take on the form of energy, Qi, rather than spirit. Their vibrational frequency decreases and the result is five different directions of movement. These movements interact with each other in endless cycles. These movements are also shown in Table 2.1. It is the various interactions of these five moving energies which cause the developmental processes of life.

Within the human energy system there are several deep meridians which form a kind of energetic 'cage'. This cage is made up of several branches of the thrusting meridian, the girdling meridian, the governing meridian and the conception meridian. The energetic cage formed by these energetic pathways is shown in Figure 2.6.

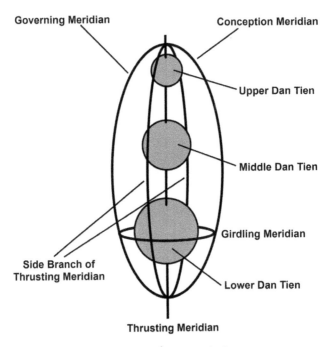

Figure 2.6: The Energetic Cage

The area of the body contained within the centre of the energetic cage is where the five energetic movements described above take place. When you have achieved a high level of skill within your internal arts practice it is possible to observe this process taking place. Within Chinese medicine these five moving energies are known as the five elements. It is these shifting vibrational patterns which dictate any predispositions you may have towards imbalances with regards to your health, personality traits and even bodily structure. This area of Chinese medicine is a whole study in its own right although the key elements of five element theory with regards to human nature and health form part of the foundational knowledge of all forms of Chinese medicine.

The movement of these five elements within the core of the energy system serve to influence the quality and nature of the Qi which flows throughout the rest of the meridian system to reach the various organs and tissues of the body which are the manifestation of the five elemental energies within the physical realm. In this way a human body is born from the original seed consciousness.

The Movement of the Five Elements

Fire Elemental Energy

The element of Fire is an expanding energy which provides warmth to the body. When in balance it pulses outwards from the core of the thrusting meridian in the area of the Heart. The warming waves of Fire energy here provide a catalyst for all the functions of the physical body as well as dictating the health of the Yang aspect of the mind and body. Figure 2.7 shows the location of the Fire elemental energy of the body and its movements.

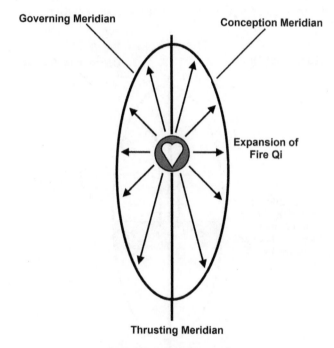

Figure 2.7: Fire Elemental Qi

In the case of an excess of Fire elemental energy there is an excess of Yang. There will likely be too much heat within the body that can damage the organs, particularly the Heart which is sensitive to Heat. The excessive heat will also cause the Shen to be disturbed which can result in manic behaviour and inappropriate laughter. People with an excess of Fire Qi are often very excitable and find it very difficult to sit still; they talk a lot and at a high speed.

A deficiency of Fire elemental energy means that the expanding waves lack force. The body does not receive enough warmth meaning that a person will feel cold. It is common for a person of this type to feel fatigued as well as emotionally flat. A feeling of sadness will often be apparent along with a dislike of social interactions.

Earth Elemental Energy

Earth elemental energy rises up from the level of the Spleen and Stomach within the energetic cage and divides as it reaches the top of the thrusting meridian. This yellow, dividing energy sits at the point of change between the other elements. It is the energy of fruition and production. Figure 2.8 shows the movement of the Earth elemental energy within the energetic cage.

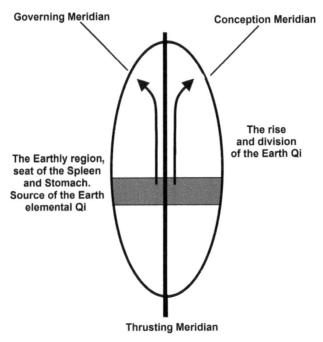

Figure 2.8: Earth Elemental Qi

If the Earth elemental energy is balanced then all the various developmental processes of the body will be healthy. The organs will be nourished and able to function as they should. This will lead to a healthy level of focus and a mind free of worries.

Any imbalances within the Earth elemental energy are often manifested within the digestive system as well as the functioning of the Spleen and Stomach. Excessively 'Earthy' people tend to be overweight and quite 'plodding' in their movements. Within Chinese medicine we often attribute an excess of Damp as being linked to an excess of Earth elemental energy and this is easy to understand if we think of the qualities of a sponge soaked in water.

A deficiency of Earth elemental energy can mean that the body does not produce energy from food as it should. The result of this can be that a person finds it difficult to gain weight as their body cannot gain nourishment from food which is a key way in which we draw in the energy of the Earth. Any imbalance within the Earth element will result in excessive worrying. It is interesting to note that in excessive type Earth patterns this worry may often be transferred onto others, resulting in smothering, overbearing behaviour, particularly towards one's own family members.

Metal Elemental Energy

The element of Metal gently contracts in towards the area of the lungs from the outside of the energetic cage. In many ways it is the opposite movement of the energy of the Fire element. When Metal energy is in balance it can be thought of as being like a reassuring hug. It serves to contain all of the other energies and draw everything in together. It helps to pull in the Heaven energy via the air we breathe as the contracting force of Metal elemental energy governs the drawing-in function of the Lungs. Figure 2.9 shows the location and movement of the Metal elemental energy within the energetic cage.

Excessive Metal energy contracts with too much strength. The result is a constriction of the energy of the body which creates a feeling of being bound up. This tightness greatly limits the expansion of the Fire energy which governs not only our ability for experiencing joy but also compassion. Excessive Metal elemental energy can result in a person being emotionally cold and quite detached. In extreme cases they can be quite ruthless in their actions. They are almost always very direct in their words and tend to lack diplomacy.

Deficient Metal elemental energy means that the contracting force is too weak; the Lungs are unable to draw in Heaven energy as they should and the physical organ of the lungs begins to weaken. This results in a lack of self-expression and a low voice. The unbound nature of the elemental energy results in feelings of sadness and an inability to 'let go' of past events which have caused hurt. It is also common for there to be issues with the large intestines. These people may be prone to feeling blocked up and suffering with constipation.

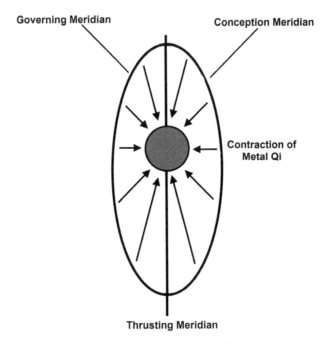

Governing Meridian

Conception Meridian

Contraction of
Metal Qi

Thrusting Meridian

Figure 2.9: Metal Elemental Qi

Water Elemental Energy

As the microcosm and the macrocosm are one and the same; the cycle of Water elemental energy within the body closely matches the water cycle within the external environment. Water elemental energy originates in the area of the Kidneys within the energetic cage. Like a still lake this energy lays dormant until the energy of the Ming Fire (see Chapter 7) provides warmth. The Water elemental energy changes to 'steam' which rises up the length of the spine through the thrusting meridian. Once the Water elemental energy hits the overhead canopy of the lungs it is cooled and begins to fall once more like rain. The Water elemental energy sinks down through the body providing moisture and governing the Yin aspect of the body. Now the cycle begins anew. Figure 2.10 shows the movement of the Water elemental energy within the energetic cage.

Excessive Water elemental energy means that there is too much energetic moisture within the body. This overacts on the Fire elemental energy restricting the expansion which is needed for warmth; the body becomes cold. These people are prone to being nervous and lacking confidence; every little aspect of life can be scary and they often fear for their own health. In extreme cases they are hypochondriacs who often spend much time going from one health practitioner to another looking for confirmation that they are indeed very sick. Sadly, because of the link between mind and body, they usually fulfil their own fears and do become seriously ill.

Deficient Water elemental energy means that the nourishing energy of the Kidneys is weakened. These people have low immune systems, weak bones and low energy levels. Along with this they are timid people who struggle to cope with life on a daily basis.

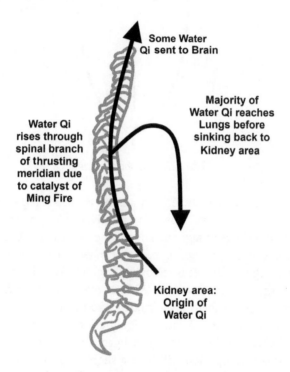

Figure 2.10: Water Elemental Qi

Wood Elemental Energy

Wood elemental energy rises straight up through the centre of the energetic cage like a plant thrusting its way up through the tarmac. This is a direct and unsubtle force that gives direction and power to all aspects of the psyche, energy system and physical body. Figure 2.11 shows the movement of the Wood elemental energy within the energetic cage.

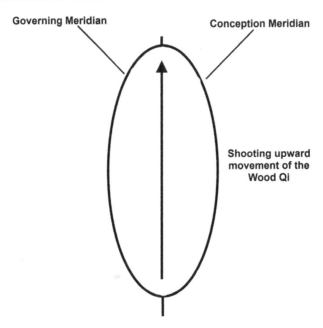

Governing Meridian   Conception Meridian

Shooting upward
movement of the
Wood Qi

Figure 2.11: Wood Elemental Qi

Excessive Wood elemental energy means that the driving force is too strong. The Wood energy moves upwards excessively like a volcano erupting. The result is feelings of rage and anger which are externally directed onto other people. It is worth noting here that anger is not necessarily seen as a negative energy which needs removing from the body; instead it is simply Wood energy with no direction. Without the guidance of directed focus it becomes anger; if focus gives guidance to the Wood elemental energy then anger is transformed into a highly creative force. Excessive Wood energy also causes the tendons and ligaments to become a little tense. The result is that a person will have a slightly 'twitchy' quality to their movements which can be quite erratic. It is difficult for them to carry out slow moving exercises such as Taijiquan or Qi Gong as they usually try to rush through the movements.

Deficient Wood elemental energy can lead to feelings of inner directed anger. The result is a sense of frustration which is often linked to feeling disempowered. The flow of Qi through the body stagnates to some degree due to the lack of driving force which can mean that a person becomes stiff and inflexible with regards to both their body movements and their thought processes.

The Physical Manifestations
of the Five Elements

As mentioned above, the five lights move into the energetic realm and become the five elemental energies which are essentially five different directions of vibrating information: Qi. From here this information condenses into the physical realm as the five vibration frequencies begin to decrease. The result is the formation of the physical organs of the body known as the Zang and Fu organs. Each element has either a Yin or a Yang physical organ attached to it with the exception of the element of Fire which also has the Pericardium and Triple Heater. Each organ has various functions attached to it; these are discussed in detail in Chapter 7. The functions of the organs are a manifestation of the movement of the element which gave birth to that particular organ. If we can understand the nature of the elemental energy which was born from one of the five lights then we can easily understand the various functional qualities of the organs associated with that element. For example: the Heart is born from Fire energy which is expansive in nature. This means that the energetic functions of the Heart according to Daoist thought rely on there being a healthy expanding movement of energy around the Heart. The expanding nature of the Heart's energy is the reason for the following functions of the Heart:

- *Pumping the Blood.* The expanding nature of the Heart's Fire Qi causes the pumping of the physical organ of the heart. As the energy moves outwards it pushes the Blood through the body to reach the various organs and tissues.

- *Directing Ying Qi into the Blood.* The key Yin function of the Heart is to direct the Ying Qi into the Blood which is then transported around the body. Ying Qi is often translated as meaning 'nutritive Qi'. This is the energy which primarily serves to nourish the organs and tissues; it nourishes because of its expansive qualities which are a direct manifestation of the expansive nature of Fire elemental energy.

- *Governing the Shen.* The Shen is discussed in more detail in Chapter 7 of this book. It sits at the centre of the consciousness within the empty space that any practitioner of meditation will be striving to connect with. It is a healthy expansion of Fire elemental Qi within the energetic realm that assists in the formation of the emptiness. It is the balance between expansion and the space within the centre of this movement that creates a harmonious dwelling for the Shen.

- *Manifesting in the Face.* The health of the Heart depends upon it not becoming too hot through an excess of Fire elemental energy which will produce damaging heat. If there is too much expansion through an excessive condition then the Heat will show in the face which will become red; the colour associated with the spiritual light which gives birth to Fire elemental energy.

Once you can understand the link between the Fire elemental movement and the functions of the Heart it will be a simple task to look at the functions of the other key organs and link them to the rest of the elements. Note that there is a much closer link between the Zang (Yin) organs and the elemental energies than there is between the elements and the Yang (Fu) organs.

Understanding the way in which the organ functions were born from the elemental movements is an essential part of the foundation knowledge which underpins the Daoist arts as well as Chinese medicine. Sadly it is an area of study which is often overlooked. Figure 2.12 summarises the link between the elemental energies and function of the Zang Fu organs.

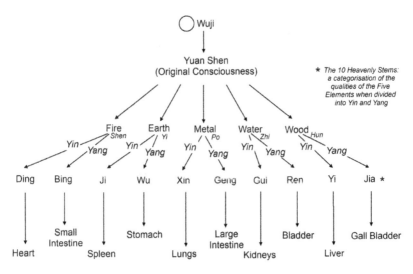

Figure 2.12: The Formation of the Organ Functions

The Balance of the Five Elemental Energies

The shifting elemental energies which are constantly interacting within the energetic cage are linked together via various relationships. These relationships ensure a healthy amount of growth, nourishment, constraint and control. In a totally balanced person these relationships would ensure that no element became too excessive nor deficient in comparison to the others. In reality there is never a fully balanced amount of all five elemental energies as they are constantly in flux. It is, however, important that through our lifestyle we ensure that they remain as balanced as possible so that illness will not take hold of our energetic system.

The various relationships of the five elemental energies can be understood through study of the diagram shown in Figure 2.13.

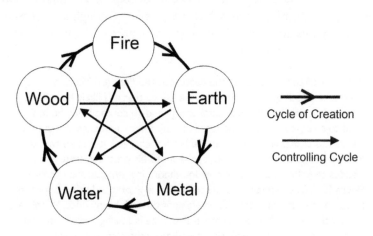

Figure 2.13: The Five Elements

The outer circle is known as the 'cycle of creation'; the inner arrows which form a pentagram shape are known as the 'controlling cycle'. While there are other cycles present within the theory of the five elements, these two are the most important. For the purposes of internal cultivation it is certainly enough to understand these two relationships well.

The Cycle of Creation (Shen)

This cycle shows how each elemental energy gives birth to the next while at the same time being born from the preceding element. For example: Fire is born from Wood and gives birth to Earth.

This cycle shows how the movement of each elemental energy reaches its peak before transforming into the next. It is a rule of Daoism that any one energy can only reach so far before it begins to transform. Yin can only reach so far before it transforms into Yang and the same rule applies to the five elemental energies. The cycle of generation can be seen within all aspects of life and development both within the body as well as within the external environment as in the case of the seasons. This is the relationship of the cyclical nature of time; the journey from birth to death before rebirth begins anew.

Within our practice we can use this relationship between the elements to our advantage. If we ascertained that we have a particular deficiency with regards to one element we would first try to change that element directly through our practice but if this did not help then we might change to working with the element which precedes it. Through strengthening the preceding element we help it to generate more of the weak element. An example is given below:

> Person A often feels cold, a little depressed and finds it difficult to express any feelings of joy. He has ascertained that it is likely he suffers from a deficiency of Fire elemental energy and so consequently he has tried to strengthen this element through his internal practice. After a few weeks it is clear that their imbalance has not changed. It is likely that the Fire elemental energy is too weak to react to his practices. Instead he decides to follow the cycle of creation theory from the diagram shown in Figure 2.13. The element that precedes Fire is Wood and so he begins to focus on strengthening the Wood element through his practice. Within a few weeks person A is feeling more elated; he is smiling more often and his hands feel warmer. Through strengthening the elemental energy of Wood he has enabled it to generate more Fire energy.

As you can see from the above example, practising according to this cycle is primarily focused on strengthening deficiencies rather than reducing excesses.

The Controlling Cycle (Ke)

The controlling cycle shows how each element exerts a restrictive influence over another element while at the same time being restricted by another. For example: Fire controls Metal while at the same time being controlled by Water.

We can use the controlling cycle within our practice if we wish to reduce an excessive element. The example below shows how this theory may be applied to our practice:

> Person B feels stressed by life. She rushes around and finds it difficult to slow down and relax. She also has a 'short fuse' and finds that she gets angry and shouts at those around her, particularly when stressed. She has ascertained that she has an excess of Wood energy. In order to calm it down she begins to focus on strengthening the Metal element. Within a few weeks she has calmed down considerably; she is more amiable to those around her and has learnt to take time out and relax so that she avoids becoming overly stressed. She did this by strengthening the elemental energy which controls Wood and keeps it in check.

Understanding these two relationships is important if we wish to understand which exercises from the five listed below to focus on when trying to bring our elemental energies into harmony.

Wu Xing Qi Gong: Balancing the Five Lights

By now you should have an understanding of the way in which the five elemental energies are formed from the seed consciousness which is passed to us from Dao via Wuji. If we are to seek any kind of internal harmony then we must first strive to bring these five elemental energies into balance. This is the first step on the path to restoring health to our energetic system. The method I present here is based upon five simple Qi Gong exercises known as the Wu Xing Qi Gong or 'Five Element Energy Exercises'. This is simple set of exercises which can be learnt by anybody within a short period of time.

For those with a strong elemental imbalance which is clear to see it is wise to practise all five of the exercises but then focus on one in particular according to either the cycles of 'creation' or 'control' from the five element diagram shown in Figure 2.13. Make sure this exercise is practiced for longer than the other four to bring your elemental environment into a harmonious state.

These exercises are the basis for the practices from the rest of the book. It is wise to build a foundation in these exercises before proceeding with any of the more advanced practice discussed in later chapters. Spend a period of a few weeks practising these each day and you will quickly build the foundation required to move onto the more advanced stages in this book.

The Wu Xing Qi Gong are as follows:

- Water Elemental Exercise
- Wood Elemental Exercise
- Fire Elemental Exercise
- Earth Elemental Exercise
- Metal Elemental Exercise

For each exercise there is a short description of the movements as well as theory as to how this balances the elemental energy associated with the exercise.

BOX 2.1: THE IMPORTANCE OF FUN

A side of training which is often overlooked, in my opinion, is the importance of having fun when practising Qi Gong. Over the course of my life I have trained with numerous different Qi Gong teachers and with various different groups. Each and every teacher has a very different approach to teaching and each class has a very different atmosphere according to the tone set by these teachers. Now in my eyes a Qi Gong class should be a light-hearted, joyous environment with much laughter and happiness. I try to foster an environment where my students study diligently and train very hard but they enjoy themselves while they are doing this. It is common for my classes to be filled with laughter and anybody who has ever trained with me will agree that my classes tend to be filled with much more noise and activity than most other classes. It is common for students coming from outside schools to be very surprised at the atmosphere in my classes. There is always a divide between those who prefer a very stern approach and those who come along and find that they prefer the light-hearted approach.

Enjoyment creates expansion and movement; these are our friends when we are training in the internal arts. Humour is a great tool when teaching as laughter creates an instant movement of Qi from the centre of the body out towards the extremities. There is much truth in the saying 'laughter is the best medicine'. It is very possible to train hard and diligently while still having fun as a group and so for this reason I encourage all those engaging in the practices within this book to laugh lots, have fun with your practices and indeed in life... It stimulates the Fire Qi.

Preparing for Wu Xing Qi Gong Practice

Begin by standing with your feet at a shoulder's width apart. Your feet should be facing forwards and your weight should be shifted so that it rests over the Yongquan (KI1) points of the feet. Suspend the head and open the spine, ensure that you have no unnecessary tension in your body while at the same time ensuring that you do not slump down as this will prevent efficient Qi flow within the body. Place the tongue on the roof of your mouth as this connects the governing and conception meridians.

Breathe deeply into the lower abdomen and gently place your mind into the lower Dan Tien area which is shown in Figure 2.14.

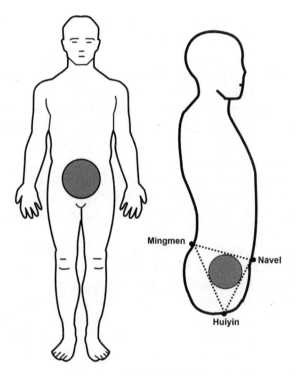

Figure 2.14: Lower Dan Tien

Empty your mind and forget all outside distractions; you should remain in this state for some time. Only when your mind is suitably still should you begin to move into the Wu Xing Qi Gong exercises.

Exercise 1: Water Elemental Exercise

Slowly bring your hands down to in front of the lower Dan Tien. Let any tension stored in the shoulders drain down through the arms and out through the finger tips. The palms of the hands (Laogong) should be facing each other as if you were holding a basketball. Make sure that the hands are not tensely forced open but at the same time they should not be limp or closed. The feeling is much like lightly stretching the tendons across the palm so that the bones can open up, a little like stretching elastic until it is only just held taut rather than stretched out to its limit.

Take your awareness from the lower Dan Tien and place it into the space between your palms. Let your focus hover here as if you are 'listening' to something very interesting taking place in the space between your hands.

Now begin to inhale and move the hands up the front of the body until they reach the height of your head. As you exhale move the hands away and back down towards the lower Dan Tien. This movement should be carried out smoothly and slowly so that you are carrying out a circular movement of the hands as shown in Figure 2.15.

Throughout this movement you should keep the hands in the original position of palms facing each other as if holding a basketball. Your awareness should also remain within the space between the hands as you carry out this movement.

Ensure that you do not raise the shoulders as your arms move upwards as this will close down the side branches of the thrusting meridian which are very important energetic pathways for the elemental energies you are working with.

Repeat this exercise at least eight times very slowly although the exact amount is not vitally important. If you are worrying too much about counting then you are not maintaining an empty mind.

This exercise matches the movement of Water elemental energy within the energetic cage as discussed previously. The movement of the awareness along with the circling motion of the hands stimulates the same directional movement on the inside of the body causing the movement of the Water elemental energy to strengthen.

Generally this exercise is practised first in the sequence, as the Water cycle stimulated through these movements helps to stir the other elemental energies.

When you have finished this exercise, return your hands to their original position in front of the lower Dan Tien with your awareness once again returning to between the palms. Remain here for a few minutes as the Water elemental energy will continue cycling for some time afterwards. After some weeks of practice you will become very aware of this movement which will likely cause the body to rock lightly forwards and backwards in time with your breath. At later stages the spine will begin to gently undulate as the Water elemental energy moves through the branch of the thrusting meridian which passes through the spinal column.

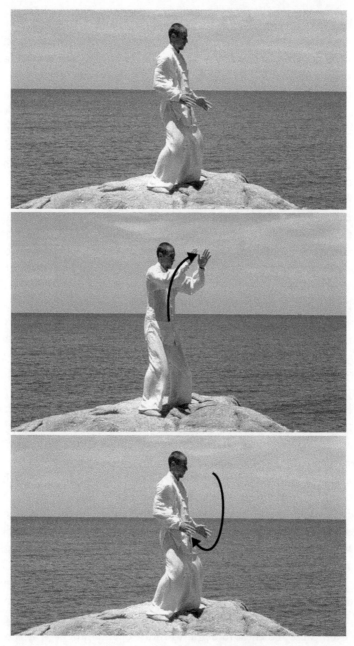

Figure 2.15: Water Element Qi Gong

Exercise 2: Wood Elemental Exercise

This exercise carries straight on from the Water elemental exercise. Inhale and raise the arms out to either side of the body with your palms facing the sky. They should rise up until they are level with the top of your head. Now fold at the elbows and bring the hands in to above your head with the palms facing downwards. Exhale as the hands move downwards until they reach the height of your hips. Continue exhaling as you move the hands around to the side of your body and then push them down towards the floor with the palms facing downwards. Figure 2.16 shows this simple movement.

As with all Qi Gong exercises, your focus is as important as the movement of your body. If the mind is allowed to wander while carrying out this exercise then it will achieve minimal results. While the hands are moving upwards your awareness should expand upwards into the Heavens. Let your mind explore the expanse above you with no limits. As your hands move in to above the head and then down towards the floor bring your awareness down through the body level with the hands until it reaches the height of the hips. The final part of the exercise involves pushing down towards the floor with your hands at your sides as shown in Figure 2.16. At this point in the exercise you should push down with your mind deep into the floor; this helps to root the Wood elemental energy.

Note that this exercise is much like the closing down movement which is common to most schools of Qi Gong. The major difference is in the use of the awareness which must be very exact. It can take some time to perfect the use of your mind in this exercise.

Once again repeat this exercise at least eight times. This exercise helps to strengthen the upwards directing force of the Wood energy as your hands lift while at the same time ensuring that it does not become too excessive as the hands move downwards in time with your exhalation.

When you have finished this exercise you should bring the hands to rest gently at your sides with the palms facing down towards the floor. Your mind should rest in your hands. Remain in this position for several minutes so that the Wood energy can continue to flow. With practice you will feel this energy moving upwards through the torso. At later stages it may even cause the chest to begin to thrust open a little as if it is being lifted from inside. This is quite normal and nothing to worry about.

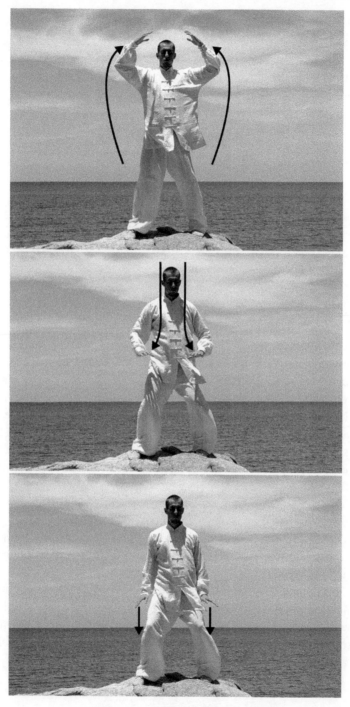

Figure 2.16: Wood Element Qi Gong

Exercise 3: Fire Elemental Exercise

From the finishing position of the previous exercise lift your hands up towards your chest and fold at the elbows. Your fingers should come together with the fingers touching and the wrists bent as shown in Figure 2.17.

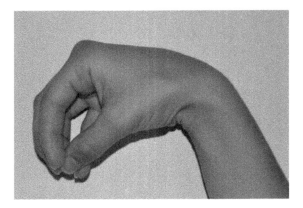

Figure 2.17: Fire Qi Gong Hand Position

In this exercise we break one of our usual rules and collapse the spine as our arms come into towards the chest. We inhale as we carry out this movement.

Next we begin to exhale and open out the body once more; our hands open out along with our arms which stretch out 45 degrees in front of us. This movement should be generated by the opening and closing of the chest and spine which then moves the arms. These two movements are shown in Figure 2.18.

This movement is then repeated at least eight times although once again the exact amount is not so important.

During the first part of the exercise, when we inhale, we bring our awareness into a meridian point in the centre of the chest known as Shanzhong (CO17) which is shown in Figure 2.19.

This point is very important for the practice as it is directly connected to the area of the body from where the Fire elemental energy begins to expand as well as being important for the regulation of our emotional centre. Our mind rests on this point as we collapse the spine and fold in our arms.

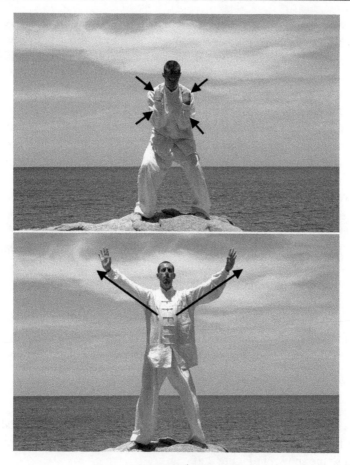

Figure 2.18: Fire Element Qi Gong

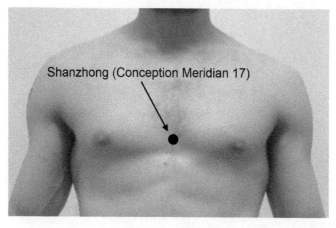

Figure 2.19: Shanzhong

As we exhale we expand the mind out in front of us as far as is possible. Let your mind fill the room if you are indoors, or if you are outside let it reach the horizon. This movement of the mind in and out along with the breathing helps to stimulate the pulsing movement of the Fire elemental energy which originates within the area of your Heart. Also, if you wish to cause the Fire energy to expand more it is useful to begin to picture something that makes you smile or laugh. Take this image that brings you merriment and keep it in your mind while performing this exercise. Stimulating joy or laughter helps to stir the Fire energy which is linked closely to this emotion.

With some practice it is possible to feel the expansion of the Fire elemental energy within your body. At later stages in the practice it is common for you to erupt into spontaneous laughter which can last for some time. If this happens then just go with it; do not try to stop the laughter as this is a sign of the Fire elemental energy moving back into balance.

When you have finished this exercise bring the hands down again into the same finishing position as the Wood elemental exercise. Have your hands at your sides with the palms facing the floor. Remain like this for several minutes with your awareness in your palms and the Fire elemental energy will continue to pulse outwards in expanding waves.

Exercise 4: Earth Elemental Exercise

From the finishing position of the last exercise bring your hands above your head and touch the thumbs and index fingers together to form the hand shape shown in Figure 2.20.

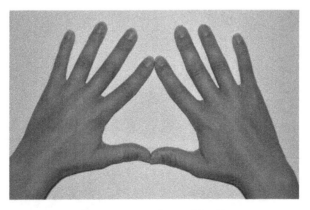

Figure 2.20: Earth Hand Position

Look upwards through the hole at the centre of this hand position. As you breathe in, fold into your legs a little and bend the arms. As you exhale straighten the arms and legs; stretch open the body and spine as you extend your focus high into the Heavens through the space between your hands. This movement is quite stretched out compared to other Qi Gong exercises and in many ways is more similar to a Dao Yin exercise than a Qi Gong exercise.

Repeat this movement for a minimum of eight times. Figure 2.21 shows this exercise being performed.

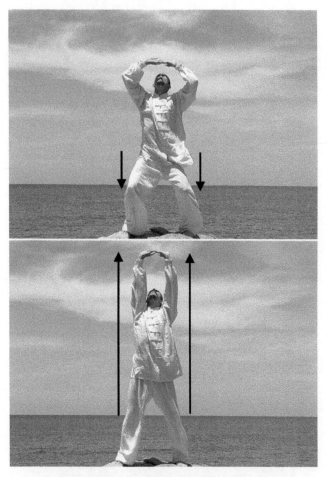

Figure 2.21: Earth Element Qi Gong Part One

There are two parts to this exercise. To perform the second part, remain in the extended position from before as if you have just finished exhaling.

Now breathe in without moving and then exhale and twist around to your left. Inhale and return to the centre before repeating the movement on the other side of your body. Throughout this movement you should keep extending your mind upwards into the sky.

Once again repeat this exercise eight times. Figure 2.22 shows the second part of the Earth elemental exercise.

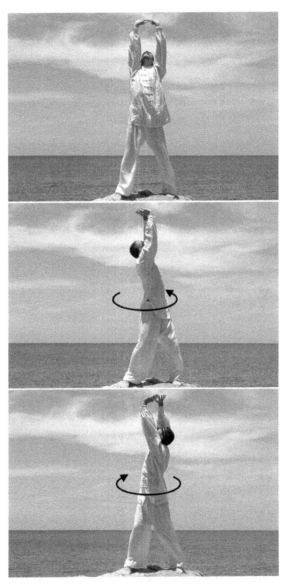

Figure 2.22: Earth Element Qi Gong Part Two

This exercise directs the rising Earth elemental energy which then divides to bring about change. The twisting movements also serve to stretch the Spleen and Stomach meridians which run along the front and sides of the torso. These are the meridians linked to the energy of Earth. Ensuring a smooth flow of information along these pathways will help to ensure that Earth Qi is flowing smoothly.

To conclude the exercise, once again bring your hands to your sides with the palms facing the floor. Rest your mind in the palms. Remain like this for a few minutes while the Earth elemental energy keeps flowing. With time you can feel the energy flowing upwards through the body before dividing.

Exercise 5: Metal Elemental Exercise

To begin this exercise, bring your hands up to your chest level with the Shanzhong point which is shown in Figure 2.19. Have the hands facing each other with your awareness resting in the space between them. As with the Water elemental exercise have your mind 'listen' to the area between the hands as if something fascinating is taking place there. This will enable your mind to connect with the Metal elemental energy in this area of the body. Remain in this position for a few minutes to establish this connection.

From here exhale and spread the arms out to your sides. You should aim to stretch out the chest so that the lungs can fully open up. Your exhalation should be through the mouth and quite fast. This will help to expel pathogens from the lungs. Have your mouth quite round and open during this part of the exercise.

Next, breathe in and bring your awareness back into the space between your hands as you return to the original position. These movements are shown in Figure 2.23.

As with the Earth elemental exercise; the Metal element Qi Gong is in two parts. Repeat part one eight times before moving onto the following movements.

In the second part of the exercise we inhale and stretch out the arms to the sides as before. Open the lungs out as you stretch open the chest. Let your mind fill the area in front of you.

As you exhale, bring the hands back in towards the centre of the chest with the palms facing each other as before. Let your awareness move in with the hands until it is once again between the hands in front of the Shanzhong point. This movement assists the gently compressing nature of the Metal elemental energy which is condensed in the chest by the above exercise. Figure 2.24 shows the second part of the Metal elemental exercise.

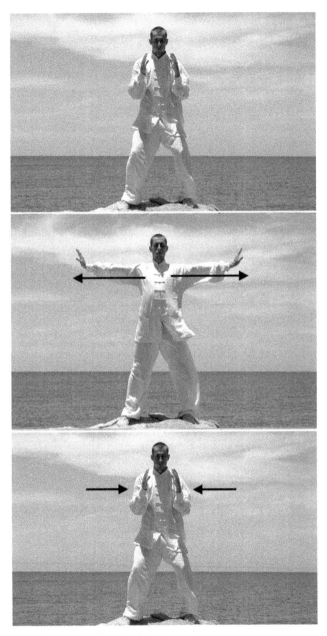

Figure 2.23: Metal Element Qi Gong Part One

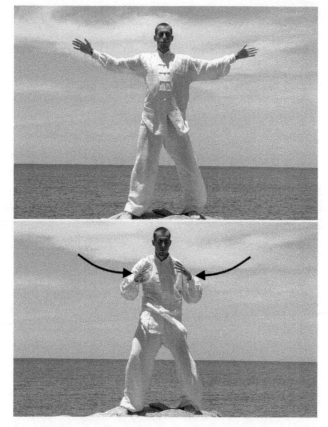

Figure 2.24: Metal Element Qi Gong Part Two

Once again, repeat this exercise eight times before concluding your practice.

Concluding the Wu Xing Qi Gong

Once you have finished your practice, stand with your feet at a shoulder's width apart and the hands hanging loosely at your sides. Bring your mind into the area of the lower Dan Tien and breathe deeply into the lower abdomen. Remain in this way for a few minutes. After this shake out the arms and legs and walk around briskly for a minute or so.

As stated above, if you have an obvious elemental imbalance then focus on the exercise which will help to bring your energetic system back into balance. Carry out each movement eight times apart from the exercise you have chosen to focus upon; carry out this exercise 16 or more times before proceeding.

The Wu Xing Qi Gong are a very simple Qi Gong set which can be learnt by anybody in a short time. There are more complex exercises which achieve similar aims but I do not believe that complicated movements can be learnt from a book alone. It is for this reason that I choose to include the Wu Xing Qi Gong here in this chapter.

If you are a practitioner of Nei Gong then please feel free to gradually integrate the various stages of Nei Gong practice into these exercises. Combining Nei Gong practice with these exercises will make them much stronger and bring better results. For more information on the practice of Nei Gong please refer to my book on the subject: *Daoist Nei Gong: The Philosophical Art of Change* (Mitchell 2011), available from Singing Dragon.

Chapter 3

HEAVENLY STREAMS

The energy that flows through us is the bond which connects the physical body to the powers of Heaven and Dao. The Heavenly Streams of the meridian system carry the vibrational information of Qi down from Heaven into our energy body. It is imperative within the study of any Daoist internal art that we become familiar with the network of meridians which were mapped out so long ago. As discussed at the beginning of the book, an experiential understanding of the meridian system is seen as the highest level of learning within the Daoist tradition but it is helpful to first have some degree of theoretical knowledge of the layout of the meridian pathways.

The Meridian System

The meridian system is spilt into two main divisions; the acquired meridians and the congenital meridians. The acquired meridians are also known as the 12 organs meridians due to their close link to the Zang Fu organs. These meridians become fully active after a person is born; prior to birth, Qi still flows in these meridians but not as strongly as through the congenital meridians which are also known as the eight extra-ordinary meridians.

These meridians work together as one harmonious system to circulate information around the body and maintain its various functions. Without the network of meridians running through the body we would be nothing but a lifeless husk. Due to their connection with the energy of consciousness which is one step above the vibrational frequency of Qi, the meridians also have strong connections to our mental faculties and emotions. As the realm of physical matter is one step below the frequency of Qi, the meridians also have a connection with the physical body, its organs and tissues.

Serving as a driving force for the Qi which flows through the meridians is the lower Dan Tien which is shown Figure 3.1. As the lower Dan Tien rotates it pushes the Qi through the energy body ensuring that information is distributed around the body as required.

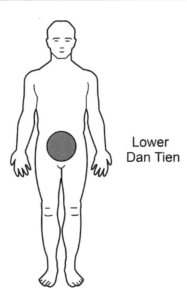

Lower
Dan Tien

Figure 3.1: The Lower Dan Tien

As the Qi passes along the length of the meridians it passes through the various Yin (Zang) and Yang (Fu) organs to provide nourishment and guiding information to govern the nature of their functioning. As well as this the organs have an effect upon the nature of the Qi which takes on various qualities. These are qualities which can be experienced at a later stage in your practice; we will discuss this at length later in the book. It is this change in nature of the Qi which passes through the organs and meridians which links the Zang Fu organs to the physical body. The result of this is that dysfunction of the Zang Fu organs can result in physical symptoms which may not, at first, seem obviously connected. These external symptoms often manifest along the length of the meridians and a skilled practitioner of Chinese medicine may use these as diagnostic signs.

The Acquired Meridians

The acquired meridians can be divided up in various ways according to different schools of thought but within this book they are generally listed according to their elemental relationships. The nature of the Qi within meridians which share an elemental relationship is similar in quality; again this is discussed later in more detail. Table 3.1 shows the elemental relationships of the acquired meridians.

Table 3.1: Elemental Meridian Relationships

	Yin Meridian	Yang Meridian
Fire	Heart	Small Intestine
	Pericardium	Triple Heater
Earth	Spleen	Stomach
Metal	Lungs	Large Intestine
Water	Kidneys	Bladder
Wood	Liver	Gall Bladder

What follows is a description of the pathway of the acquired meridians of the body as well as a very brief overview of the benefits of accessing each meridian.

Heart Meridian

The Heart meridian originates internally within the physical organ of the heart and the area of the middle Dan Tien. From here it moves internally to the axilla where it emerges on the exterior of the body and travels down the posterior border of the medial aspect of the arm to the tip of the little finger. Internally a branch of the meridian descends through the diaphragm into the small intestines which are paired elementally with the Heart. A second internal branch ascends through the throat to connect with the eyes which are also linked elementally with the Heart. Figure 3.2 shows the pathway of the Heart meridian.

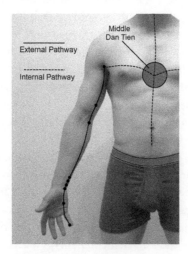

Figure 3.2: The Heart Meridian

The information which travels within the Heart meridian has a close relationship to the 'space' where the Shen resides within human consciousness. For this reason it can be utilised within Daoist practices to connect with the spirit and bring harmony to the mind. The middle Dan Tien sits within the area of the Heart as shown in Figure 3.3.

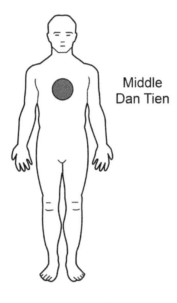

Middle
Dan Tien

Figure 3.3: The Middle Dan Tien

The origin of the Heart meridian sits within the physical organ of the heart and the energetic area of the middle Dan Tien which governs the ebb and flow of our emotions. For this reason the Heart meridian may be utilised within Daoist practices to calm the emotions and bring about mental harmony. Although each organ is linked to a different aspect of our emotional self, the Heart meridian sits within the area of the middle Dan Tien where these individual emotions are experienced. This means that the Heart has a close relationship to the emotional aspect of all the other organs of the body.

The expanding energy born from the spiritual light of Fire circulates within the energetic cage of the congenital meridians. It is at the origin point of the Heart meridian that it connects with the Qi of the Heart meridian and moves down into the Heart and Pericardium meridians. It is for this reason that these two meridians may be utilised within Daoist practices to regulate the Fire elemental energy of the body as well as the feelings of inner warmth and joy which are governed by this energy.

Small Intestine Meridian

The Small Intestine meridian originates on the little finger close to the finish point of the Heart meridian. It ascends the ulnar aspect of the back of the hand and then travels up the posterior aspect of the arm to the area of the shoulder blade where it zigzags across to connect with the governing meridian at the 7th cervical vertebrae before running over the shoulder to the supraclavicular fossa. Here it ascends the throat and travels across the face to the cheek and the ear. Internally, a branch descends from the supraclavicular fossa through the physical organ of the heart down to the small intestines. Figure 3.4 shows the pathway of the Small Intestine meridian.

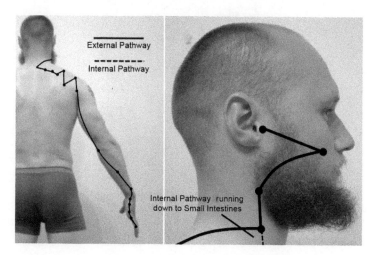

Figure 3.4: The Small Intestine Meridian

The Small Intestine meridian can be accessed and used to treat imbalances within the small intestines as well as pain or tightness in the shoulders due its location. As well as this it connects to the emotional aspect of our consciousness that deals with the ability to understand right from wrong. Balancing the energy within this meridian will allow a person to tackle any consciousness issues around this area.

The Small Intestine meridian runs along the shoulders and the medial aspect of the elbows. These areas are particularly susceptible to the negative effects of the energetic pathogen of Wind which is often the precursor to illness. For this reason, the Small Intestine meridian may be accessed by Daoist practitioners to expel Wind and prevent the further progression of many diseases which are based upon the effects of external pathogens.

Pericardium Meridian

The Pericardium meridian originates within the physical organ of the heart where it connects to the membranous sack of the pericardium which encases the heart. From here an internal branch descends deep inside the body to connect with the lower chamber of the Triple Heater with which it is elementally paired. A second branch moves to the chest where it emerges lateral to the nipple. This external branch now descends the medial aspect of the arm to conclude on the middle finger. Figure 3.5 shows the pathway of the Pericardium meridian.

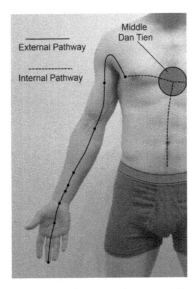

Figure 3.5: The Pericardium Meridian

Like the Heart meridian, the Pericardium meridian has a connection to the energetic location of the middle Dan Tien. This connection means that the energy within the Pericardium has a close connection to the emotions.

The Pericardium's main function is to protect the sensitive organ of the Heart from excess Heat. This Heat is often generated internally by excessive emotional disturbances which, without the protection of the Pericardium, would be very detrimental to the functioning of the Heart. For this reason the Pericardium meridian may be accessed by Daoist practitioners to expel excess Heat from the body, especially at the point of Laogong (PC8) which sits at the centre of the palm. This is a key point of the body for expelling Heat based pathogens and in effect acts as a kind of energetic exhaust pipe.

Triple Heater Meridian

The Triple Heater meridian originates at the tip of the ring finger. From here it flows across the dorsum of the hand to ascend the lateral aspect of the arm to the shoulder. It travels across the shoulder to the supraclavicular fossa where is ascends the neck, encircles the ear and then concludes at the lateral end of the eyebrow. An internal branch from the supraclavicular fossa descends through the pericardium to the lower energetic chamber of the Triple Heater. Figure 3.6 shows the pathway of the Triple Heater meridian.

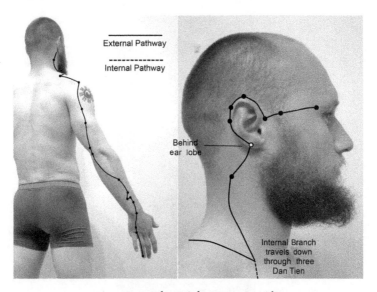

Figure 3.6: The Triple Heater Meridian

The Triple Heater meridian connects the three Dan Tien and the energetic chambers which they govern. This meridian is primarily accessed by Daoist practitioners who wish to adjust the functions of the three Dan Tien and the energetic substances which they govern.

The Triple Heater meridian can also be accessed to improve the flow of energy in general around the entire body via a couple of key points on the arm and hand; these are important points which are often underestimated with regards to their value. These points are discussed later in further detail.

Spleen Meridian

The Spleen meridian originates at the tip of the big toe where it travels along the medial aspect of the foot and the posterior border of the tibia. The meridian travels past the knee to the abdomen which it ascends to the anterior aspect of the chest. Here it sharply descends to conclude on the lateral midline at the height of the diaphragm. An internal branch enters the stomach and spleen where it ascends through the throat to enter the tongue. Figure 3.7 shows the pathway of the Spleen meridian.

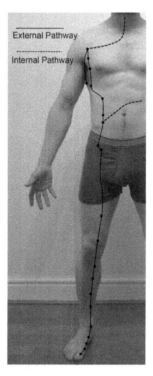

Figure 3.7: The Spleen Meridian

The Spleen meridian is considered the key meridian of the Earth elemental energy which flows through the energetic cage of the congenital meridians. It is the main meridian accessed to adjust the balance of the Earth elemental energy.

The Spleen is considered the creator of the acquired energy within the body due to its function of drawing essential energy from food and drink which transforms into the acquired Qi of the body. This Qi is also connected to the health of the Blood and so accessing this meridian can help to adjust any imbalances within the Qi and Blood of the body.

Damp is a difficult internal pathogen to clear from the body; it is the Spleen which is accessed to help clear Damp from the body. This is because the Spleen's function, when strengthened, will help to transform the turbid fluids of Damp into a more refined substance which can be processed more effectively by the body.

The Spleen meridian can also be accessed to treat most digestive disorders and any pains which may exist along the length of the Spleen meridian.

Stomach Meridian

The Stomach meridian originates externally directly inferior to the eye. From here it travels along the line of the jaw to reach the lateral aspect of the forehead. From Daying (ST5) it descends the throat to the supraclavicular fossa and descends the chest along the line of the nipple to the abdomen and anterior aspect of the leg. The meridian continues to descend the leg, travel across the foot and then concludes at the tip of the second toe. Figure 3.8 shows the pathway of the Stomach meridian.

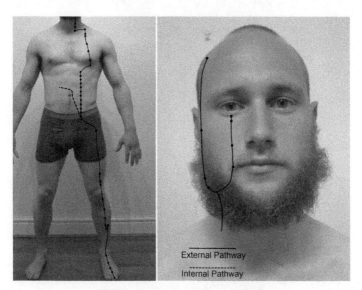

Figure 3.8: The Stomach Meridian

The Stomach meridian is the Yang meridian which conveys the Earth elemental energy around the body. It can be accessed to treat pain and any energetic obstructions along the line of the meridian which travels the length of the entire body.

The Stomach meridian is very effective for treating any issues around Damp obstructions in the body so arthritic conditions can be helped by accessing the Stomach meridian. A few key points on the legs can also be accessed to govern the quality of Qi in the body; this will be discussed in detail later in the book.

Lung Meridian

The Lung meridian originates within the physical organ of the lungs. From here an internal branch descends through the diaphragm to enwrap the large intestines which are elementally linked with the Lung meridian. A second internal branch ascends through the throat where it turns towards the lateral aspect of the chest where it emerges externally. The external pathway of the Lung meridian descends along the medial aspect of the arm to conclude on the thumb. Figure 3.9 shows the pathway of the Lung meridian.

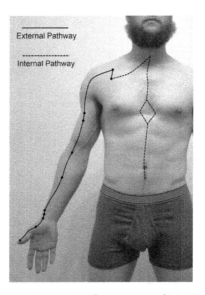

Figure 3.9: The Lung Meridian

The Lung meridian is the main pathway through which the elemental energy of Metal travels. It can be accessed to adjust the level of Metal elemental energy which is circulating within the energetic cage of the congenital meridians. The meridian can also be accessed by Daoist practitioners to affect the physical organ of the lungs as well as the throat and chest.

Addictive behaviours can be treated through the use of the Lung meridian along with the Kidney meridian. This is due to the connection between the Lungs and the Po which can also be connected with to calm the mind and treat spiritual disorders.

The lungs are delicate organs which are easily affected by external pathogens; for this reason we may access the Lung meridian to expel external pathogens from the body if they are caught early enough and have not travelled deeper into the body.

Large Intestine Meridian

The Large Intestine meridian originates at the tip of the index finger. It travels along the index finger and then passes along the anterior aspect of the arm to the shoulder. From here the meridian moves to the supraclavicular fossa where it ascends the neck to the cheek before travelling past the mouth where it concludes at the opposite side of the nose near the nostril. An interior branch descends from the supraclavicular fossa through the physical organs of the lungs. It concludes within the large intestines. Figure 3.10 shows the pathway of the Large Intestine meridian.

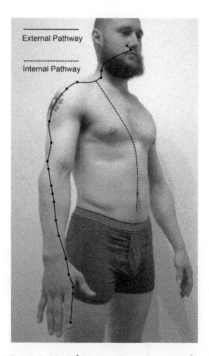

Figure 3.10: The Large Intestine Meridian

The Large Intestine meridian can be accessed to treat pain and energetic obstructions along its length, particularly on the shoulder and around the lateral aspect of the elbow. It also has a strong effect on those who have difficulties with the physical organ of the large intestines as well as on the emotional aspect of letting go. Those who cannot rid their mind of some past hurt or grudge may access the energy of the Large Intestine meridian to help them move on with their lives.

Kidney Meridian

The Kidney meridian originates on the sole of the foot at the very important point known as Yongquan (KI1). It travels behind the medial malleolus up the medial aspect of the leg to the upper thigh where it enters the body and connects with the base of the spine. This internal branch travels up through the lumbar vertebrae to move through the physical kidneys to exit the body once more on the lower abdomen. From here the Kidney meridian travels up the anterior of the body to end on the upper chest. The internal branch near the kidneys continues to ascend through several organs including the liver and lungs before it concludes at the base of the tongue. Figure 3.11 shows the pathway of the Kidney meridian.

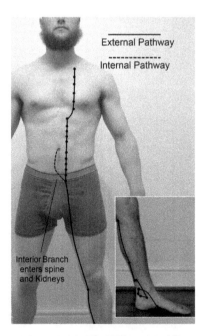

Figure 3.11: The Kidney Meridian

The Kidney meridian is a very commonly accessed meridian. It helps to govern the quality of the Jing and restore energy to those who are particularly depleted. This helps to strengthen the back and knees as well as draw in a stronger connection to the vibrational force of the planet.

The Kidney meridian can also be utilised to help with imbalances of the uterus.

Because of the Kidneys' relationship to the Lungs, it is common to access the Kidney meridian to strengthen the rooting of Heaven energy in the body which will help to strengthen the Lungs.

This is also the key meridian to be accessed when seeking to rebalance the Water element within the body.

Bladder Meridian

The Bladder meridian originates at the inner canthus of the eye. It ascends to travel across the head where it descends to the occiputs. Here it divides into two branches which travel down the length of the back parallel with the spine. Both these branches reconnect on the legs where they travel along the lateral aspect of the foot to conclude on the lateral aspect of the little toe. An internal branch connects the Bladder meridian into the physical organ of the brain. Figure 3.12 shows the pathway of the Bladder meridian.

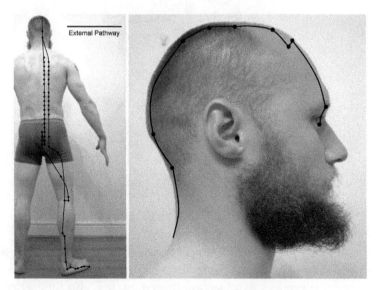

Figure 3.12: The Bladder Meridian

The Bladder meridian can be accessed to clear energetic blockages which may sit along the line of the Bladder meridian which runs along the entire length of the back. Due to the location of the Shu points it can also be used to treat weakness within any of the Zang Fu organs of the body.

Liver Meridian

The Liver meridian originates on the big toe. From here it travels along the dorsum of the foot and then along the medial aspect of the leg to the groin where it travels around the genitalia and then ascends the abdomen. An internal branch runs through the gall bladder, liver and diaphragm. Within the torso it spreads out into the hypochondriac region before ascending through the throat to the eyes. From here an internal pathway ascends to the vertex of the head. Figure 3.13 shows the pathway of the Liver meridian.

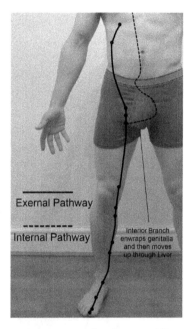

Figure 3.13: The Liver Meridian

The Liver meridian is the main meridian which provides a pathway for the Wood elemental energy. It is the key meridian accessed to help govern the emotional energies of anger and frustration. It is also the meridian accessed to prevent Liver energy rising which can give birth to migraine type headaches.

Energetic blockages along the length of the Liver meridian usually manifest within the inside of the legs and around the groin area; these can often be cleared through use of the Liver meridian.

Gall Bladder Meridian

The Gall Bladder meridian originates at the outer canthus of the eye. From here it travels to behind the ear before sharply returning back over the head to above the eye. Another sharp turn sees the meridian travelling back over the head to the base of the neck before it runs anterior to the shoulder to the lateral aspect of the thorax. The Gall Bladder meridian zigzags down the side of the body to the lateral aspect of the leg where it continues down to the lateral aspect of the leg to the fourth toe. An interior branch enters the body where it travels through the liver and gall bladder which are elementally linked. This pathway continues down to the hips where it reconnects with the external pathway of the meridian. Figure 3.14 shows the pathway of the Gall Bladder meridian.

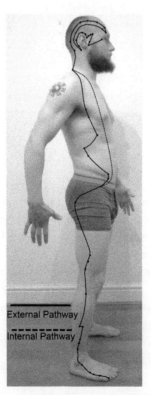

Figure 3.14: The Gall Bladder Meridian

The Gall Bladder meridian can be accessed to treat energetic blockages anywhere along its length which means that it governs blockages along the entire lateral aspect of the head and body; common areas for blockages to appear. Many temporal headaches are linked to energetic blockages along the length of the Gall Bladder meridian.

Any physical injury can be helped by accessing the Gall Bladder at several points which connect with the energy governing the tissues and tendons of the body.

Congenital Meridians

The eight congenital meridians transport vital energetic information which helps in our development prior to birth. After birth the energy here slows down considerably and the congenital meridians serve mainly as reservoirs for the Qi which later reaches the acquired meridians. Through internal practice we seek to reverse this process and restore a healthy degree of movement in the congenital meridians; this is one of the key stages of internal development within the Daoist practice of Nei Gong. The various 'small water wheels' of Qi which Daoism practices focus on are circulations of information which take place within the congenital meridians.

The energetic cage which contains not only the three Dan Tien but also the five elemental energies is formed from the congenital meridians, and is of particular importance for the practices contained within this book.

Governing Meridian

The governing meridian originates within the energetic area of the lower Dan Tien; within women it also starts within the physical organ of the uterus. From here it descends to the perineum where it then ascends the posterior midline, travels over the head and concludes on the upper lip. An interior branch connects the upper governing meridian with the brain. Figure 3.15 shows the pathway of the governing meridian.

The governing meridian has several important points which can be accessed to help strengthen the function of the Kidneys (via the Ming Fire), nourish the brain and lift the consciousness. It also has a strong effect on the health of the back.

Those seeking to work with the lower Dan Tien through practices such as Nei Gong can also help the process by accessing certain points on the governing meridian.

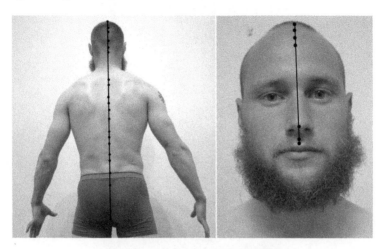

Figure 3.15: The Governing Meridian

Conception Meridian

It is important to note that the pathway of the conception meridian according to Daoist theory differs from contemporary Chinese medicine theory; the flow is understood to travel in the opposite direction. Such differences are common within a tradition which spans several centuries; different masters followed different conceptual frameworks. From my own personal experience the primary flow of energy within the conception meridian does indeed run downwards.

According to Daoist theory the conception meridian continues from the concluding point of the governing meridian where it descends the anterior midline to the perineum where it internally connects with the lower Dan Tien and the uterus in women. The governing and conception meridians, in effect, form one circular meridian which encircles the entire body. Figure 3.16 shows the pathway of the conception meridian.

Accessing the conception meridian can enable direct access to the lower Dan Tien and the seats of Jing and Qi within the body. It is also the main meridian through which the uterus is accessed and all gynaecological imbalances can be regulated through contact with this meridian.

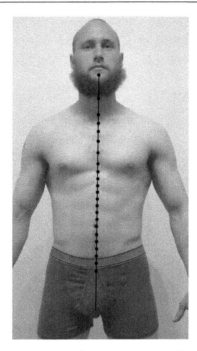

Figure 3.16: The Conception Meridian

Thrusting Meridian

The theory of the thrusting meridian also differs between the Daoist school of thought and contemporary Chinese medicine. According to Daoism the thrusting meridian has several branches.

- The first branch runs through the centre of the body from the crown of the head to the perineum. This branch connects the three Dan Tien and governs the flow of all energy through the core of the energy body. It is an important meridian within Daoist Nei Gong and meditation practices as it serves as a kind of spiritual antennae through which contact with higher levels of consciousness can be made once a person reaches a high enough level of attainment.

- A second branch runs through the centre of the spine. This branch moves energy from the area of the kidneys up into the brain. It also governs the energetic strength of the spine.

- Two side branches run through the left and right sides of the chest and abdomen. These serve to regulate the balance of Yin and Yang within the body.

- Extra branches run through the centre of the arms and legs; they ensure that congenital energy reaches the extremities.

Figure 3.17 shows the various branches of the thrusting meridian.

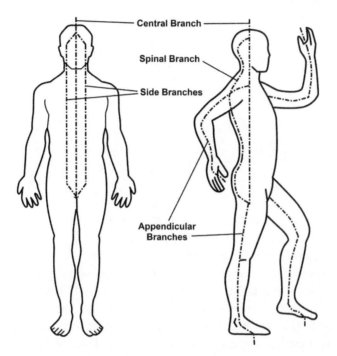

Figure 3.17: The Thrusting Meridian

Accessing the thrusting meridian has a profound effect upon the spiritual aspects of a person's nature due to the conversion of Jing to Qi to Shen which takes place within this meridian along with the three Dan Tien. The vertical pole of this meridian is particularly important and connecting with this element of the thrusting meridian can give the instant experience of the realm of emptiness which sits at the centre of the energy body. This is explored in greater depth towards the end of this book.

The thrusting meridian is often known as the 'sea of blood'. For those with imbalances which manifest as excessive bleeding, particularly menstrual bleeds, accessing this meridian can be useful.

Girdling Meridian

The girdling meridian is unique in that it is the only meridian to run horizontally through the body. Figure 3.18 shows the pathway of the girdling meridian.

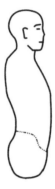

Figure 3.18: The Girdling Meridian

The function of the girdling meridian is to enwrap the lower Dan Tien and help it to rotate efficiently. It also serves as a form of energetic compass. Those with an imbalance in the girdling meridian will have a tendency towards a poor sense of direction; they will easily get lost. Accessing the girdling meridian can help to rebalance this issue. It also has connections to various functions associated with organs in the lower abdomen but for all intents and purposes it is easier to access these organs via their own individual meridians. It is unlikely that we access this meridian through our internal practice very often.

Yin and Yang Linking Meridians

The Yin and Yang linking meridians serve to regulate the flow of Qi throughout the rest of the meridians. They are rarely used in the practices outlined in this book and are included here only for completion purposes. Figure 3.19 shows the pathway of the Yin and Yang linking meridians.

Yin and Yang Heel Meridians

Within Daoist internal practices the Yin and Yang heel meridians help to pull excess energy away from the head where it could be dangerous if it collected too rapidly. In essence this means they work much like the earthing wire on an electrical circuit. We do not use them very much in the practices outlined within this book as they are fairly self-regulating but they have been included here for completion purposes. Figure 3.20 shows the pathway of the Yin and Yang heel meridians.

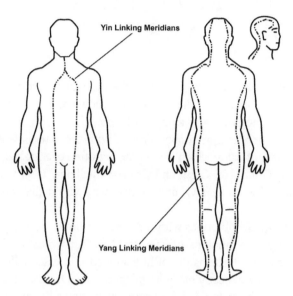

Figure 3.19: The Yin and Yang Linking Meridians

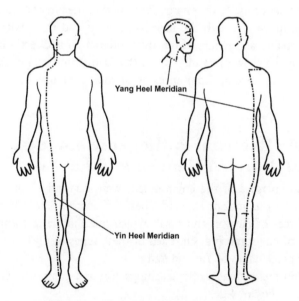

Figure 3.20: The Yin and Yang Heel Meridians

CHAPTER 4

THE MOVEMENTS
OF HEAVEN

In the previous chapter we looked at the individual meridians and how
they relate to the organs. This is essential knowledge in the study of any
of the Daoist internal arts along with the information covered in this
chapter: the meridians as communicators with the external environment.
This is an area of study which is integral, but often overlooked, within the
areas of Qi Gong, Nei Gong and Chinese medicine. It takes the various
movements of a person's Qi and places them within the context of the
wider universe.

The energetic vibrations within the human body are directly reflected
in the energetic vibrations of the world within which we live. As we
have already stated, the nature of human matter is, essentially, emptiness.
Human beings are mostly made up of space. The Daoists understood this
and saw how the energy of the environment flowed through this space
meaning that we are little more than conduits for the movement of Qi
which surrounds us. As the energy flows within the environment it enters
the body, moves through the meridian system and then exits meaning
that the quality and nature of our own internal Qi is directly influenced
by the Qi which we live in. This is the Daoist understanding of how
imbalance can develop from an external source. Figure 4.1 summarises
this concept.

The Six External Pathogenic Factors,
Fluctuations of Heaven and Earth

The main energies of the environment were categorised into six main
headings by the ancient Daoists. These six energies are a combination
of the forces of Heaven and Earth which intermingle to form different
qualities of environmental Qi. Each of these types of Qi is formed from
different percentages of Yin and Yang.

Within the ancient Daoist teachings, Yin and Yang were symbolised
as shown in Figure 4.2.

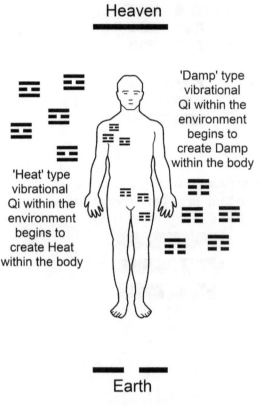

Figure 4.1: Human Conduits

Figure 4.2: Yin and Yang

Yin is represented by a broken line while Yang is a solid line. This is the basis for the classic text of the Yi Jing or *Classic of Changes* (see the glossary) which is a key classical text within Daoism and an integral part of any Daoists study.

The Yin and Yang lines are initially organised into groups of three. The resulting images are known as Trigrams or Gua. Examples of Trigrams formed entirely of Yin and Yang lines are shown in Figure 4.3.

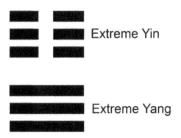

Figure 4.3: Yin and Yang Gua

The extreme manifestations of Yin and Yang within our realm of existence are Heaven and Earth so we can represent these as shown in Figure 4.4.

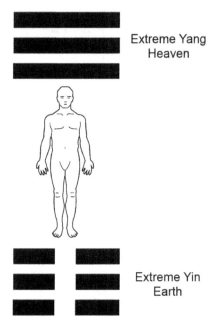

Figure 4.4: The Placement of Heaven and Earth

Human beings now sit at the empty space between Heaven and Earth, extreme Yang and Yin. It is within this space that the various interplays of Yin and Yang also take place.

When Yin and Yang are combined into their various different combinations, the Trigrams shown in Figure 4.5 are created. These six symbols represent the different ways in which the energies of Heaven and Earth may intermingle and manifest.

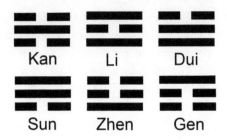

Figure 4.5: The Interactions of Heaven and Earth

The resultant six energies each have their own characteristics and qualities which, like everything else, manifest on different levels. Although these manifestations take place, once again on a spiritual, energetic and physical level, matters are also complicated as these energies manifest differently both within and outside of the body. For this reason I have summarised the different qualities and manifestations of the six Trigrams that exist between Heaven and Earth in Table 4.1.

Table 4.1: The Six Key Trigrams between Heaven and Earth

	Li	Gen	Dui	Kan	Sun	Zhen
Quality	Warming	Stagnating	Drying	Freezing	Moving	Moving
Element	Fire	Earth	Metal	Water	Wood	Wood
Climate	Heat	Damp	Dryness	Cold	Wind Heat	Wind Cold
Pathogen	Fire	Damp	Dryness	Cold	Wind	Wind
Season	Summer	Late Summer	Autumn	Winter	Spring	Spring

Heaven and Earth interact with each other to produce different environmental energies; one manifestation of these is the climate. Contemporary Chinese medicine practice lists six different external climatic states which may have an effect upon our health. These are as follows:

- Wind
- Cold
- Damp
- Dryness
- Heat
- Summer Heat

Essentially, Heat and Summer Heat are two different manifestations of the same climatic influence. Summer Heat is a more extreme version of Heat. It is also possible to divide Wind into the two different types: Wind Heat and Wind Cold. For this reason, when looking at the climate from a Daoist perspective according to the Trigrams the list becomes:

- Wind Heat
- Wind Cold
- Cold
- Damp
- Dryness
- Heat

A discussion of each of these six climatic energies now follows with its corresponding Trigram.

The Li Trigram (Heat)

Figure 4.6 shows the Trigram arrangement known as Li which manifests primarily as Heat within the environment.

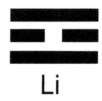

Figure 4.6: The Li Trigram

The Li Trigram shows one Yin line in the centre with Yang lines above and below it. This is representative of the energy of Li moving out from the centre. The Yang movement of Qi spreads out in expansive waves. The result of this is an energy with warming qualities which, if in excess, can lead to overheating.

When this energy manifests as a pathogen within the body it creates internal heat which expands and moves upwards. This is a Yang pathogen so it usually causes the Yang aspect of an organ or the body in general to become excessive while the Yin aspect becomes deficient.

In extreme cases the Heat affects the Heart which is linked to it by the element of Fire. If this happens then the Blood can become hyperactive due to the Heart's Yang function of propelling the Blood. The following is a list of classical signs associated with the pathogen of Heat:

- A dislike of being in a warm environment
- Fever
- Sweating
- Confusion
- Thirst

The Gen Trigram (Damp)

Figure 4.7 shows the Trigram arrangement known as Gen which manifests primarily as Damp within the environment.

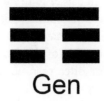

Gen

Figure 4.7: The Gen Trigram

The Gen Trigram depicts two Yin lines topped by a Yang line. This represents the fact that this energy is Yin in nature and tends to move downwards. The Yin Qi is literally sinking down towards the planet. It is thick and heavy in nature. When it manifests within the environment it is a muggy energy which is stifling.

When Gen manifests within the body as the pathogen of Damp it is similar in nature to its environmental energy. Damp is heavy and constricting. It is the energy of stagnation and obstruction. A body filled with the energetic pathogen of Damp will always feel heavy and the person will often feel very tired. Since it is a 'sticky' pathogen it is often quite difficult to shift. The following is a list of classical signs associated with the pathogen of Damp:

- A feeling of being heavy
- Dull body aches
- Tired muscles
- Swelling of the joints and body
- Sudden digestive upsets

The Dui Trigram (Dryness)

Figure 4.8 shows the Trigram arrangement known as Dui which manifests primarily as Dryness within the environment.

Dui

Figure 4.8: The Dui Trigram

The Trigram of Dui is depicted as being two solid Yang lines below one broken Yin line. This is representative of Yang energy (Heat) affecting the Yin energy above which it causes to dry up. When it manifests within the environment it is a climate with little moisture; dry air that is difficult to breathe in. Interestingly we have now created our own artificial environments which exist outside of the seasons through the invention of air conditioning and more often than not this creates an environment with the Dui energy of Dryness.

When Dui manifests within the body as a pathogen it is drying in nature. The Yin fluids of the body become deficient resulting in dry skin and cracked lips. The following is a list of classical signs associated with the pathogen of Dryness:

- Dry cough
- Dislike of a cold environment
- Fever
- Dry skin, particularly around the nose and mouth

The Kan Trigram (Cold)

Figure 4.9 shows the Trigram arrangement known as Kan which manifests primarily as Cold within the environment.

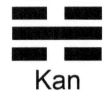

Kan

Figure 4.9: The Kan Trigram

The Kan Trigram shows one solid Yang line surrounded by two broken Yin lines. This shows that the energy of Kan is contracting in nature as the Yin energy moves in to squeeze the Yang energy within its centre. When this energy manifests within the environment it is cold.

When Kan becomes the pathogen of Cold it constricts the energy of the body causing it to 'freeze'. Cold is Yin in nature and so tends to impair the Yang energy of the body which means that a person's body temperature will drop.

Prolonged periods of the pathogen of Cold being held within the body will also result in stagnation of Qi and Blood due to Cold's constricting nature; the pathogen literally prevents everything from moving. The following is a list of classical signs associated with the pathogen of Cold:

- Stiffness

- Muscles' contraction

- Dislike of cold weather

- Cold limbs and body temperature

- Possible diarrhoea

The Sun Trigram (Wind Heat)

Figure 4.10 shows the Trigram arrangement known as Sun which manifests primarily as Wind Heat within the environment.

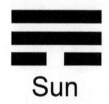

Sun

Figure 4.10: The Sun Trigram

The Trigram of Sun depicts two solid Yang lines atop one broken Yin line. This shows a Yang, warming energy which is prone to sudden change as a new Yin energy arises from below it. Two lines the same atop one of the opposite nature always indicates a tendency towards change. This is the energy of Sun which manifests within the environment as a warm breeze or, at its most extreme, a tropical hurricane.

Within the body, Sun manifests as Wind Heat. This is a fast moving, Yang pathogen which tends to attack the upper body first. It brings pain and discomfort within the body that moves very suddenly, usually through the meridians. This pathogen can suddenly arise and then swiftly move on or change into one of the other pathogens.

The following is a list of classical signs associated with Wind Heat:

- Dislike of a warm environment
- Sore throat
- Runny nose
- Headache
- Fever
- Pain that moves suddenly throughout the body

The Zhen Trigram (Wind Cold)

Figure 4.11 shows the Trigram arrangement known as Zhen which manifests primarily as Wind Cold within the environment.

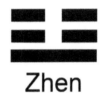

Zhen

Figure 4.11: The Zhen Trigram

The Zhen Trigram is depicted as having two broken Yin lines above one solid Yang line which is bringing sudden change to the lines above it. It is the opposite of the Sun Trigram and so has a relationship to Sun of mirroring its qualities.

While Sun is manifested within the environment as a warm breeze, Zhen is a cold, biting wind. When Zhen becomes a pathogen within the body it is Wind Cold. Like Wind Heat, this energy is swift moving and quick to change but this energy brings with it the qualities of Cold as well, primarily contraction.

The following is a list of classical signs associated with Wind Cold:

- Dislike of a cold environment
- Sore throat
- Runny nose
- Sneezing

- Headache
- Pain that moves suddenly throughout the joints

A Note on Wind

It is often said within Chinese medicine that 'all pathogens may begin with Wind'. Wind is quick to change and the most unpredictable of the pathogens. For this reason it is likely that Wind Heat and Wind Cold may quickly develop into one of the other pathogens when it enters the body. Contrary to what you might expect, Yin and Yang may change into each other quite rapidly so Wind Cold may turn into the pathogen of Heat while Wind Heat may transform into the pathogen of Cold; such is the unpredictable nature of Wind.

Energetic Change across the Seasons

Just as the movement of the weather is a manifestation of the energies of Heaven and Earth interacting, so are the seasons. The cycle of spring, summer, autumn, winter and back to spring is due to the effects of Yin and Yang cycling through the five elements. This cycle of birth, development and death reflects the will of Heaven and reflects the constantly changing nature of Yin and Yang which Daoists seek to understand experientially.

This process of change can be shown with the Trigrams which enable us to map out the shifts in Yin and Yang Qi which take place throughout the year. Having this conceptual framework of something which is essentially very abstract enables us to understand the patterns which exist within the cosmos that surrounds us. When a form of energy shifts into another form we can map this out with the Trigrams. When a Trigram changes, one of two things can happen: either one line of the three changes to its opposite form or the entire Trigram reverses to its mirror image. If only one line changes then this shows a subtle change which is gradual and smooth. If the entire Trigram reverses to its opposite then there has been a sudden and dramatic change. Figure 4.12 shows this change of Trigrams according to the cycle of the seasons.

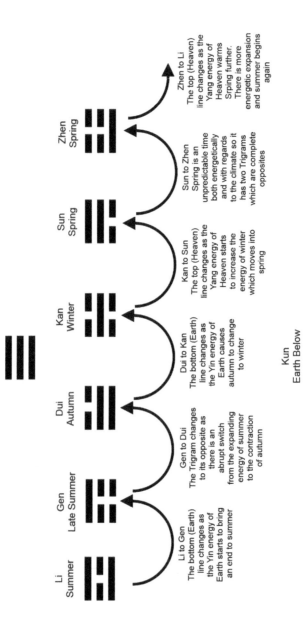

Qian
Heaven Above

Kun
Earth Below

Li
Summer

Gen
Late Summer

Dui
Autumn

Kan
Winter

Sun
Spring

Zhen
Spring

Li to Gen
The bottom (Earth) line changes as the Yin energy of Earth starts to bring an end to summer

Gen to Dui
The Trigram changes to its opposite as there is an abrupt switch from the expanding energy of summer to the contraction of autumn

Dui to Kan
The bottom (Earth) line changes as the Yin energy of Earth causes autumn to change to winter

Kan to Sun
The top (Heaven) line changes as the Yang energy of Heaven starts to increase the energy of winter which moves into spring

Sun to Zhen
Spring is an unpredictable time both energetically and with regards to the climate so it has two Trigrams which are complete opposites

Zhen to Li
The top (Heaven) line changes as the Yang energy of Heaven warms Srping further. There is more energetic expansion and summer begins again

Figure 4.12: The Seasons and the Trigrams

This dominance of different energies throughout the seasons of the year is also reflected within the inner environment of the body. The energies which surround us also affect the way in which the Qi within our body acts; it governs which of our internal organs is energetically dominant. It is worth noting that within each season we will have more of a tendency towards the pathogen that is dominant during that particular season although we can contract any pathogen at any time of the year. Refer back to Table 4.1 to see which pathogen is associated with each season.

It is also worth noting that as the energy of our organs cycle in time with the seasons they each have a peak and a trough with regards to their energetic power. Each organ is strongest during the season it is linked to and then weakest during the following season. This reflects the fact that each organ's energy will move into a Yang state and peak shortly before it moves into a Yin state and dips in strength. This cycle matches the sequence of the five elements which any practitioner of the Daoist arts should be familiar with. It is summarised in Table 4.2.

Table 4.2: Seasonal Strengths of the Organs

	Spring	Summer	Late Summer	Autumn	Winter
Strongest Organs	Liver Gall Bladder	Heart Small Intestine	Spleen Stomach	Lungs Large Intestine	Kidneys Bladder
Weakest Organs	Kidneys Bladder	Liver Gall Bladder	Heart Small Intestine	Spleen Stomach	Lungs Large Intestine

With regards to practice, it means that it is more difficult to strengthen the energy of an organ when it is in its deficient season of the year and difficult to reduce any excesses in an organ when it is in its season of dominance. For example: Kidney deficiency is difficult to improve during spring while an excess of Stomach energy is difficult to reduce during late summer.

External Invasions

The six environmental energies are a natural part of the Qi which surrounds us. They are rarely still and can change from day to day although different seasons will lend themselves towards having different qualities depending upon which of the six environmental energies are dominant. They should have little effect on the human energy system providing that the environmental energy is not too extreme or the body's internal energy is not too weak. The balance between environmental energy and body's internal energy dictates whether or not the vibration frequency of the outside world will begin to have a detrimental effect upon the vibration frequency of the energy within the meridian system. Figure 4.13 summarises this concept.

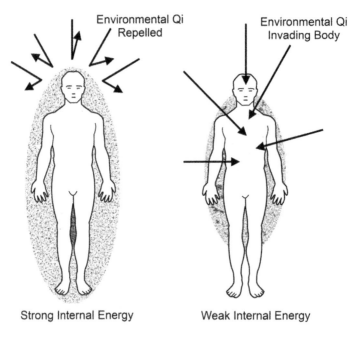

Figure 4.13: Environmental Qi and Internal Qi

If the body's own internal energy is weak for whatever reason then the environmental energy will enter and the symptoms outlined above will begin to manifest as the body's Qi is changed in quality. For example:

In the dead of winter when temperatures drop below freezing, those with poor quality internal energy will find that Cold begins to change the nature of the Qi within their body. This is called a 'Cold invasion' and will likely manifest as stiff joints, cold limbs and possibly loose bowels. This is the beginning of imbalance from an external source and it is likely that this will develop into an illness if the Cold is not expelled in time.

The Six Divisions

We have already discussed how the meridians of the body can be categorised according to their elemental relationships. These give us an understanding of how the different energies of the meridians relate to each other and hold each other in balance. There is a second key method of categorising the meridians which is known as the six divisions. These are six pairings of the 12 acquired meridians, which enables us to understand the nature of the meridian system's relationship to the world around us. These six divisions are named: Tai Yang, Shao Yang, Yang Ming, Tai Yin, Shao Yin and Jue Yin. Each of these six divisions is linked to a pair of meridians as shown in Table 4.3.

Table 4.3: The Six Divisions of the Meridians

Division	Meridians	Environmental Qi
Tai Yang (Greater Yang)	Bladder and Small Intestine	Cold
Shao Yang (Lesser Yang)	Triple Heater and Gall Bladder	Wind Heat
Yang Ming (Shining Yang)	Stomach and Large Intestine	Dryness
Tai Yin (Greater Yin)	Lung and Spleen	Dampness
Shao Yin (Lesser Yin)	Heart and Kidney	Heat
Jue Yin (Terminal Yin)	Pericardium and Liver	Wind Cold

As you can see from the table, each of these six divisions also has an associated environmental energy. In some schools of thought, Wind Heat is replaced with Summer Heat and sometimes the order of the six divisions appears differently. These are differences that have come about from a tradition which was largely passed down orally for centuries and reflects the personal understanding of the different masters who held the knowledge at different times. It is often the case that argument breaks out between followers of different conceptual frameworks but this shows a misunderstanding of the organic nature of change within the Daoist arts. The differences are only minor and experience will show that they all have their merits in practice.

Six divisions can be confusing at first, especially for those who are more familiar with the five elemental way of categorising the meridians. Five element theory is focused more on the organ relationships of the meridians while six divisions is focused more on the way in which the meridians interact with the outside environment. Let us look at each of these six divisions individually.

Tai Yang (Greater Yang)

The Tai Yang meridians of the Bladder and Small Intestine form one unit as shown in Figure 4.14. They are considered the meridians with the strongest relationship to the external environment.

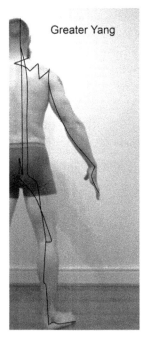

Figure 4.14: Tai Yang

As you can see from Figure 4.14, the Tai Yang meridians run along the length of the back and the posterior aspect of the shoulders. They govern the most Yang aspect of the physical body and are the key meridians involved in protecting the body from external Cold invasions. In China it is considered of vital importance that people wear scarves and hats as soon as the weather is even the slightest bit cold and the lower back must be covered at all times. The aim of this is to cover the Tai Yang meridians which will otherwise be prone to Cold invasion. It is common for this Cold to be transferred along the line of the Bladder meridian resulting in a tight, aching back.

Shao Yang (Lesser Yang)

The Shao Yang meridians of the Triple Heater and Gall Bladder form one unit as shown in Figure 4.15. At this point in the meridian system, the external energy of Tai Yang, which relates strongly to the external environment, is beginning to slow and transform ready to move in towards Yang Ming. For this reason, Shao Yang is sometimes known as the conversion aspect of the Yang divisions.

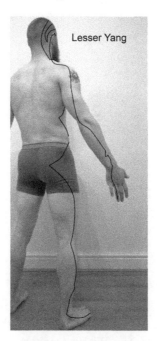

Lesser Yang

Figure 4.15: Shao Yang

The Shao Yang meridians are easily affected by Wind Heat which means that rapidly changing energy (Wind) within the environment has produced the result of Heat within these meridians. This Heat produces stagnation which is the enemy of Shao Yang. Both Shao Yang meridians are accessed through various Daoist practices to clear heat from the body. If the Wind Heat is transferred through the Gall Bladder meridian it often creates a tension type headache in the temporal region.

Yang Ming (Shining Yang)

The Yang Ming division is comprised of the Stomach and Large Intestine meridians as shown in Figure 4.16.

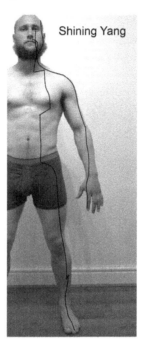

Figure 4.16: Yang Ming

The Yang Ming aspect of the meridian system is the point at which Yang begins to transform into Yin. Within Daoist philosophy Yang can only expand so much until it reaches a peak and has to change into Yin. This process is matched within Daoist alchemical practices whereby Jing (Yin) is transformed into Shen (Yang). When this Shen (Yang) reaches its peak it is transformed into the emptiness of Dao, stillness (Yin). Within the meridian system it relates to the environmental energy of Dryness.

Each of the six divisions is said to have a different amount of Qi and Blood flowing through it as shown in Table 4.4.

Yang Ming is unique in that it has neither more Blood nor Qi; it has an even abundance of both. It is for this reason that the Yang Ming meridians are often accessed to rebalance any problems that have arisen within the Qi and Blood of the body. This abundance of Qi and Blood makes Yang Ming fairly moistening; the Stomach and Large Intestine organs do not like to be excessively dry as this weakens their function and so dryness transmitted along the Yang Ming meridians into the interior of the body can cause disharmony this way. Yang Ming also has a strong relationship with the next in the six divisions, Tai Yin which has to be kept in balance with Yang Ming to maintain the correct balance of moistness with dryness.

Table 4.4: Qi and Blood in the Six Divisions

Division	Qi	Blood (Xue)
Tai Yang	Less	More
Shao Yang	More	Less
Yang Ming	Much	Much
Tai Yin	More	Less
Shao Yin	More	Less
Jue Yin	Less	More

Tai Yin (Greater Yin)

The Tai Yin division is comprised of the Lung and Spleen meridians which form one unit as shown in Figure 4.17.

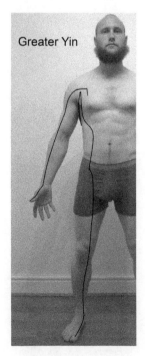

Figure 4.17: Tai Yin

Tai Yin is the point at which Yang energy begins to transform into Yin; it sits at the cusp of change and is pivotal in the balance of the energies of Heaven and Earth. The Lungs draw in the Heaven energy via our breathing while the Spleen converts energy from the food which we eat; food is one of the key ways in which we draw in the energy of the Earth.

The Tai Yin aspect has a close relationship with the Yang Ming aspect which precedes it sequentially. Even the organs are linked elementally. The Lung (Tai Yin) is linked with the Large Intestines (Yang Ming) and the Spleen (Tai Yin) is linked with the Stomach (Yang Ming). These organ relationships reflect the balance of Dryness against Damp as the Tai Yin aspect does not like Dampness, the environmental Qi it is prone to invasion from. Tai Yin is responsible for enabling the body to adjust to Dampness in the environment and if it is not able to do this due to weakness then Damp will enter the body via these meridians and be transferred internally to the organs of the Lungs and Spleen.

Shao Yin (Lesser Yin)

The Shao Yin aspect of the meridian system is comprised of the Heart and the Kidney meridians. It is shown in Figure 4.18.

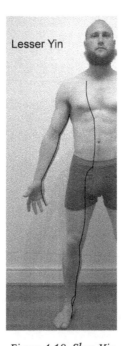

Figure 4.18: Shao Yin

The Shao Yin aspect of the meridian system enables our energy system to communicate with the Heat within the external environment. It is comprised of the Heart and the Kidneys which have a close relationship via the Fire and Water balance of the body. Figure 4.19 shows this relationship between the Heart and Kidneys.

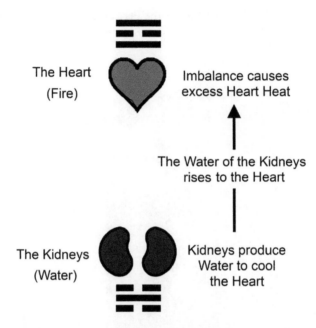

The Heart
(Fire)

Imbalance causes
excess Heart Heat

The Water of the Kidneys
rises to the Heart

The Kidneys
(Water)

Kidneys produce
Water to cool
the Heart

Figure 4.19: Fire and Water Balance of the Heart and Kidneys

The Heart is a delicate organ which is considered the most important of the organs within Chinese medical thought; it is often named the monarch of the organs. The Heart does not like to be excessively hot and for this reason it is protected by the Pericardium which helps to vent excess Heat prior to it attacking the Heart. As the Heart becomes hot the Kidneys generate more Water energy, essentially a vibration frequency which helps to neutralise the information which is causing damage to the Heart. This gradually drains the Kidneys which can become deficient through the process of producing this Water Qi. It is interesting to note that the Heart is caused to heat up by any emotional disturbances and poor diet as well as by external Heat invasions. This means that excess emotional disturbances and eating poor quality food will also drain the Kidneys which are vital for our vitality and continued good health.

The environmental energy of Heat can invade the Shao Yin aspect of the meridian system resulting in excess Heart Heat as the imbalance is transferred inwards.

Jue Yin (Terminal Yin)

The Jue Yin division is comprised of the Pericardium and Liver meridians which work together as one unit as shown in Figure 4.20.

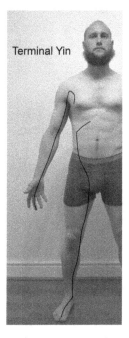

Figure 4.20: Jue Yin

Jue Yin is the most Yin of the six divisions. It is the period of stillness and rest that is in complete opposition to the extreme movement of Yang energy. This manifests within the organs of the Liver which stores the Blood when the body is in rest and the Pericardium which helps the hyper activity of the Heart, due to emotional stress, come to rest. This calming influence which the Pericardium exerts upon the Heart helps to protect it from extreme imbalances developing.

Jue Yin is most damaged by the environmental energy of Wind Cold or, in many forms of Chinese medicine, Wind of any sort. In order to understand how this energy relates to Jue Yin we should understand the nature of Wind. Wind is a fast moving change in the nature of the energy of the environment, this is in direct contrast to the nature of Jue Yin which likes to be calm and still; it is for this reason that Wind and especially Wind Cold attacks the Jue Yin division of the meridian system. The Liver is also said to be prone to giving rise to an internal form of Wind. This is due to the fact that the Blood stored in the Liver (Jue Yin has more Blood than Qi, remember) helps to strengthen Jue Yin preventing Wind Cold from entering the body. If the Blood is deficient within Jue Yin then there is little protection from the environmental energy of Wind which will get into the body.

Experiential Study

By now you should have an understanding of the core theories of how the seed consciousness gives birth to the energy system via the five spiritual lights; perhaps you have already experienced the movements of these five elemental energies through practice of the Wu Xing Qi Gong. You should also have an understanding of the meridian system, how it relates to the physical body and how it connects to the environmental energies, Heaven and Earth. Further theory needs to be explored including the nature and functions of the organs of the body and signs for when these are in a state of imbalance. This theory is covered later in the book as now it is wise to begin exploring the energy body for yourself; it is time to gain a direct experience of the nature of the energy body.

CHAPTER 5

ENTERING THE STREAM

Intellectual learning can only take you so far, tangible experience is the way to truly understand the nature of human Qi. This is the stage of 'entering the stream'. In times past the Daoist sages sat in quiet contemplation exploring every inch of their own energy body. Over time they mapped out the entire system which they had travelled through with their own minds, honed through years of meditation practice. This invaluable knowledge was preserved and passed on in charts and books which were studied by their disciples alongside the same inner exploration which had uncovered these energetic pathways in the first place. Within this book so far there has been a presentation of the basic theory of the meridian system and how it relates to the outside world; now comes the second part of the puzzle – connecting the mind to the meridian system.

In order to connect with your energy body we need to first train the aspect of our consciousness which is most easily directed by our mind. This is the Yi, our awareness, focus and intention. Unlike the ethereal spirits of Shen and Hun which lay close to the vibrational frequency of Heaven or the dense energies of Zhi and Po which lay rooted within the matter of the physical world, the Yi sits at the border between physicality and the spiritual realm. As the consciousness manifestation of the Earth element it sits at the centre of the elemental cycle, the most balanced of the elements with regards to Yin and Yang characteristics. Figure 5.1 shows the centred nature of the Yi.

It is our Yi which dictates whether or not we will be able to successfully focus on a task which we have set our self, or whether we will be distracted by our wandering thoughts.

The key to controlling the Yi is learning how to link it to the movement of Qi and our breathing. These three can come together as one unit to enable us to begin to 'enter the stream' and learn how to connect with the energetic realm. This is a basic process which forms an important part of the foundation for arts such as Qi Gong although many people neglect to spend enough time on this important part of the practice.

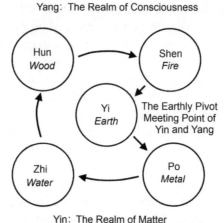

Figure 5.1: The Yi, the Earthly Centre

Breath, Yi and Qi

Our breathing sits at the threshold between our energy body and our physical body. The way we breathe has a strong effect on both the physiological processes of the body and also the movement of our Qi through the meridians. For this reason it can be thought of as a kind of translator which enables the energy body and physical body to communicate. Within Chinese culture this link is well understood and the character for Qi can also mean 'air'. The process of breathing also has a calming influence upon the mind; this calming process takes place as the movement of the breath calms the spirit of the Lungs, the Po, which in turn settles the Yi. Figure 5.2 summarises the link between breath, Po and Yi.

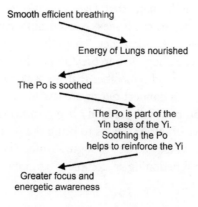

Figure 5.2: Breathing and Consciousness

If the breathing is efficient then the Qi will be led smoothly through the body. Much like a gentle gust of wind passing over the surface of a still lake, the movement of the breath causes a gentle wave through the meridians preventing stagnation from developing. Too little wind and there are not enough waves. Too forceful a wind and the waves become choppy and the water's surface rough; this can be seen in those who breathe too forcefully, they have a rough, choppy feel to their energy flow. This also creates stagnation which begins to have a detrimental effect upon the energy of the Liver which is related to the quality of Qi flow through the body; the result of this is a build-up of feelings of frustration and annoyance.

Qi and Yi are both middle level vibration frequencies. Qi has Shen above it and Jing below; Yi has Hun and Shen above it and Po and Zhi below. This means that their frequencies are of a similar nature and can be used together as one unit. This is very important within Daoism as according to the philosophy which underpins all Daoist arts, the mind has the power to change reality. This is a viewpoint which is fairly constant throughout many Eastern spiritual traditions and a truth which has become more apparent to me the deeper I have moved into my own practice. If we are able to train our Yi to a high level then by virtue of the intention of our thoughts we are able to adjust the way in which Qi flows. It is interesting that, since Qi is a universal energy which binds the microcosm of our body to the macrocosm of the environment, this means that powerful enough intention is strong enough to change the energy of the world we live within. Truths such as this place the human mind in a very powerful position.

Regulating the Breath

It is important to understand that Daoism never aims to change the natural order of things; instead it seeks to ascertain what the natural order is and realign itself with this order. This ethos applies to all that we do including the regulation of our breathing. Throughout the process outlined below you should remember that we seek to observe a process that is taking place and connect our awareness to it. This connection of mind and natural process will gradually begin to bring about a positive change as the power of our Yi begins to bring the process into line with the flow of energy which moves through all life. The only reason that we are not already functioning in complete harmony with this force is because we have become disconnected from it. Unity brings harmony while disconnection brings imbalance. If you seek to consciously hurry or force the processes outlined within this book then you run the risk of making a mistake and increasing the level of disharmony present within your inner environment. Daoism is a tradition of going with the flow.

Those who already have a breathing practice such as Sung breathing will be able to add the following practice without it clashing. Connecting the Yi to the breath and the Qi will serve to complement any existing breathing practice you already have.

The process of regulating the breath for the practice in this book is fairly simple and split into three key stages:

1. Listen to your breathing

2. Observe the change

3. Harmonise with the Yi

These three stages are outlined below.

Listen to Your Breathing

It is quite amazing that although people breathe from birth to death, they rarely take the time to take a look at this process. It is one of our most common bodily functions and yet one we generally choose to ignore. Unless a person engages in some kind of internal practice they often take the process of breathing totally for granted. Strangely I have even met practitioners of the internal arts who took their breathing for granted.

Observing the breath is best carried out early in the day when you first wake up or in the evening prior to sleep providing you are not too tired. These are generally much calmer times of day for most people although you will usually find what times suit you best after practising for a while. Go to a quiet place where you will not be disturbed and begin to practise for around 10–15 minutes at a time. As you move deeper into this process you will most likely find that your practice extends into an hour or more; this should be allowed to happen naturally, never force it.

For those who are comfortable with sitting practices such as meditation, the first position shown in Figure 5.3 is useful for this practice. If sitting for long periods of time is uncomfortable then lay down as shown in the second image in Figure 5.3.

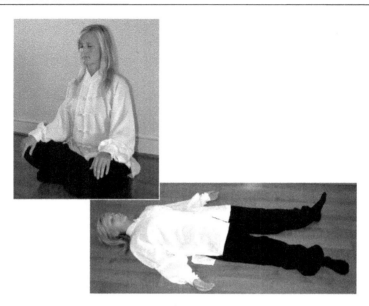

Figure 5.3: Breathing Practice Positions

Try to let all outside concerns leave your mind. At first this will be difficult and countless trivial thoughts will begin to race through your head, pictures will pop up and worries about imagined things you have to do will begin to try and disturb your practice. This is fine, just let it happen. Do not try to stop any of this mental chatter; instead just remain calm with your eyes closed and wait for the mind to calm down. It will most likely take some time but eventually it will quieten down so that you may begin to focus properly upon your practice.

When you feel ready, begin to listen to the breathing. When I teach I tend to use the word 'listen' rather than 'watch', 'feel' or any other descriptive word. Experience has shown me that when people watched their breathing they subconsciously began to imagine a great many things. People with a tendency towards image-based minds would picture a wonderful array of things, all of them beside the point. Once I began telling my students to listen to the process taking place they stopped producing so many images and began to get far more useful results. This process of listening to what is taking place is obviously not with the ears but rather with the mind. It is also the descriptive word for this process which is used by the Chinese when they teach this practice.

Begin to work through the following process:

- Listen to the movement of air as it enters the nostrils.

- Listen to this movement of air as it goes down into the lungs.

- Listen to the way in which your lungs fill with air and the diaphragm moves downward into the abdominal cavity.

- Listen as the lungs empty and the air begins to move back out through the nostrils.

- Repeat this process.

Keep your level of focus fairly light. Remember that the idea is only to observe, not to change. Keep with this practice until you can comfortably listen to this process taking place.

Observe the Change

The process of connecting your awareness to your breathing will bring about union of breath and Yi. It may take some time to become totally aware of the movement of air as you breathe in and out but persevere and you will find it a very clear process.

From here it is a natural process to begin developing an awareness of the nature of your breathing. You will most likely notice one of several different things:

1. The length of time it takes to inhale and exhale may not be equal. Some more advanced breathing techniques actually aim to adjust the timing of inhalation and exhalation but regular breathing should be even in length. This reflects the balance of Yin and Yang being cycled through as Heaven energy is drawn into the body through inhalation.

2. The breathing may not be smooth. Either the inhalation or exhalation will feel as though it judders. This is usually caused by tension which is stored in the intercostal muscles or stagnated Wood energy which is sat upon the diaphragm.

3. The breathing may wheeze. Perhaps this is something which you have not previously noticed as it may be fairly quiet. This is traditionally a sign of phlegm building up in the lungs due to stagnation of the Qi of the Lungs.

4. Short inhalation and exhalation which feels rushed and fairly weak is also common. This is sign of a weak energetic relationship between the Lungs and the Kidneys.

5. You may begin to cough as your awareness focuses upon the breathing. This is a sign of the Lung energy being weak; it is often accompanied by a feeling of anxiety.

6.   A metallic taste may begin to appear in the mouth. This is sign of excessive toxic Qi within the energy system which the Lungs are attempting to expel.

There is no need to attempt to adjust these imbalances within the breathing process. Instead focus upon the breathing as before; continue to listen to the process taking place and continue your practice every day. The above signs are marks of being out of sync with the flowing energy of Dao which runs through life. Continue to observe the above processes taking place and gradually your breathing will begin to change.

It will grow deeper, slower and smoother as even this early stage of practice begins to rebalance the state of your body. Even if you never progress past this point in your practice you will still draw great benefit from simply sitting/laying and listening to your own breathing.

Harmonise with the Yi

To link your awareness to the movement of your breathing you must continue with the stage before this until any major imbalances in your breathing have smoothed themselves out. You do not need perfection though, improvement is enough. If you have managed, for example, to slow your breath down and deepen it but you still have a slight tightness that will not go away then do not worry. It is likely that this tightness is caused by an imbalance somewhere deeper inside the energy system and you will not be able to correct this until a later stage in your practice.

Place your hands in the position shown in Figure 5.4. The palms should be facing up straight towards the sky.

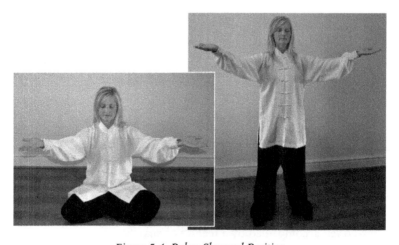

Figure 5.4: Palms Skyward Position

Open out the fingers until you feel them slightly stretch. They should not be excessively forced open but at the same time they must not be limp as both of these will inhibit Qi flow. This is a rule that applies to the entire body during any internal arts practice. Excessive tension creates sputtering, erratic Qi flow which leads to hyper-function of the organs while being limp or collapsed creates stagnation as the Qi flow slows down. The general rule is that your body should always aim to be relaxed but gently stretched open as this ensures smooth Qi flow which is not inhibited by tension in the muscles or stopped by closed joints.

Place your awareness into your palms. There is no longer any need to focus on listening to your breathing; by now it should be of a high enough level that it should take care of itself. Let your awareness gently rest this way in the hands while you continue to breathe deeply. After some time you will begin to become aware of a tangible sensation appearing in the palm of your hands. This sensation is much like the tide washing up and down the beach; on each exhalation you will be able to feel a wave of tingling and warmth flow across the palm. As you exhale this flow of Qi will subside much like the sea washing back down the beach. The reason for this is that if you place your awareness (Yi) onto an area of the body it will begin to lead the Qi. It has become an observation of mine over the years that Qi does not actually move that quickly. This was a big surprise to me as, for some reason, I had assumed that it moved rapidly through the body. In fact it moves in a very casual, 'I won't be hurried' way through the meridians. As my awareness increased over the years I began to find that Qi also moves like this outside of the body within the environment. It is only during times of disharmony that it picks up pace both within and outside of the body. For this reason it will take a little time for the Qi of your body to reach the location of your awareness which is sat in your palms. The more you practise this, the quicker your Qi will understand what it is supposed to do and so the lag time will decrease.

As you exhale Qi moves outwards from the centre of your body and as you inhale Qi moves in towards the centre of the body. This is the same for everybody. As your breathing slows down and connects with your awareness it will begin to connect also to your energy body. The combination of Yi and breath will begin to bring the movement of Qi under your control.

Stay at this stage for some time getting used to the movement of Qi being led by your awareness down to the hands. As with the stage of listening to your breathing, keep observing this process and over time it will grow in intensity. It is wise to stay at this stage and keep practising like this until you have a very strong feeling for the way that Yi and breath move your body's Qi.

Once you have managed to complete the above stage you will have managed to harmonise your breathing and train the Yi to such a stage that it is possible to move onto connecting with your meridians.

The Nature of Meridian Points

Along the length of the meridian pathways lie numerous meridian points. There are 360+ classical points which are sat along the main meridian pathways plus countless extra points which are still being added to by experienced Chinese medical practitioners. The traditional understanding of an acupuncture point is a location on the body where the Qi of the Zang Fu organs is passed to the external surface of the body or vice versa. The Chinese characters commonly used for acupuncture points can be translated as meaning 'cavity' and 'transportation'; if we look at these two characters we will get a good idea of the definition of a meridian point from a Chinese medical perspective.

When looking at the meridian points from a perspective of utilising them within our internal practices we can look at them another way: as information converters. It is at the meridian points that the Qi of the body communicates with the outside world; some acupuncture points take a stronger role in this process of internal/external communication than others and we will discuss these in further detail later. The meridian points enable the meridians, which flow beneath the surface of the skin, to transfer information out of and into the body. It is through these points that the six environmental Qi can pass into the meridians affecting the internal climate of the body. Certain meridian points have a closer relationship to the outside world than others and all of the points are inter-related in a complex web which is a lifetime study in itself.

Within our practice we can use the meridian points to convert the frequency of our mind to that of the energy of the meridians. If we can learn how to place our focused awareness onto specific areas of the meridian system and combine this with our breathing then the frequency which our mind is tuned into will change. The result is that the mind is able to perceive the meridian system as easily as it perceives the physical body. This will give us a tangible feel for the meridian which over time will refine until we are able to distinguish between different energies within that meridian as well as being able to find blockages and disruptions of the flow of Qi along the length of the meridian. With time the mind learns how to remain tuned into the meridian system and this practice is no longer required. After many years of practice I am now able to tune into my meridian system very easily; the sensation of my meridians is as tangible for me as the sensation of my physical body. Some people who I have met naturally have this ability to some degree but in my experience it was enhanced by these practices. The majority of people who I teach, however, do not have the ability to feel their own energy body and so the skill must be trained.

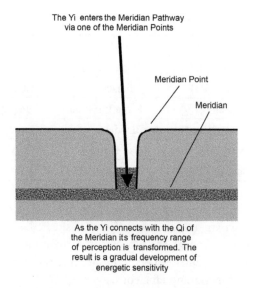

Figure 5.5: Connecting with the Meridian System

Like weaving thread through a small hole we must learn to direct our awareness into the meridian points so that the frequency may be converted allowing the meridian to open up to us. Figure 5.5 shows this process.

Yuan Source Points

Meridian points are categorised into different types according to which meridian they are on and their individual properties. One such category is the Yuan 'source' points, which are important points when attempting to connect with the individual meridians.

Each of the 12 acquired meridians have a Yuan source point which is classically understood to have an effect upon the congenital energy of each individual meridian. These points are some of the first points discussed within the Chinese classical text of the Ling Shu (Spiritual Pivot) and to this day are considered of the utmost importance in the treatment of any internal disease. Each of the Yuan source points also has a connection to the energy of the Triple Heater via various tiny branches which come off of the main meridians to move deep into the body. Within Chinese medical practices such as acupuncture these points are utilised to bring nourishment from the original essence circulated by the Triple Heater into the meridian which has become weakened. The Yuan source points are listed in Table 5.1.

Table 5.1: Yuan Source Points

Meridian	Source Point	Meridian	Source Point
Heart	Shenmen (HE7)	Small Intestine	Wangu (SI4)
Spleen	Taibai (SP3)	Stomach	Chongyang (ST42)
Lung	Taiyuan (LU9)	Large Intestine	Hegu (LI4)
Kidney	Taixi (KI3)	Bladder	Jingu (BL64)
Liver	Taichong (LV3)	Gall Bladder	Qiuxu (GB40)
Pericardium	Daling (PC7)	Triple Heater	Yangchi (TH4)

The location of these points is shown in Figure 5.6. Each point sits around the areas of the wrists, ankles or feet. They are situated at areas which are always moving a great deal, the movement at these joints stimulates the function of the Yuan source points to ensure that the original essence of each meridian is functioning efficiently.

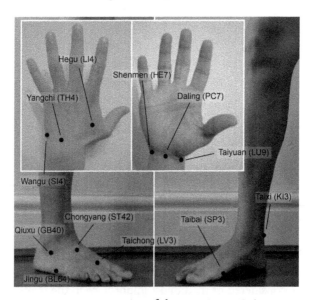

Figure 5.6: Location of the Yuan Source Points

It is wise to spend some time familiarising yourself with the location of these points. The lists at the end of this book give more accurate descriptions of these points to ensure that you can locate them easily. Spend some time massaging the points and getting to know them as they are going to be the main entry points for your practice. The only exception is the Yuan source point of the Kidney meridian as I have found that there is an easier entry point on the base of the foot: Yongquan (KI1), which we will discuss shortly.

Connecting with the Lung Meridian

The meridians are connected with one at a time. In my experience I have found it easiest to connect with the Lung meridian first. The majority of students who I have taught also found this to be the case so I would suggest that you start there. The Lung meridian runs along the arm as shown in Figure 5.7.

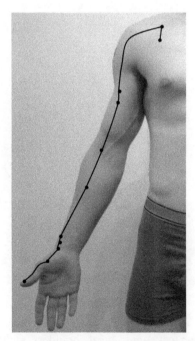

Figure 5.7: External Pathway of the Lung Meridian

As with the rest of the meridians on the arm, the Lung meridian runs closer to the surface between the elbow and the fingers/thumb. This is the easiest part of the meridian to connect with and so we will start there.

First, locate the Yuan source point of the Lung meridian; ensure that the location is accurate and then massage the point with your thumb for a couple of minutes to ensure that you have its position locked in your mind. The massaging of the point also ensures that the Qi in this area is stimulated which will make the next stage fairly easy.

Next, stand in the position shown in Figure 5.8. This position is often known as Zhan Zhuang or 'standing post' posture. The Qi Gong system of Zhan Zhuang has its own series of stages to work through which are very complex but for the purposes of this exercise we are just using the position as it ensures that the meridians of the body are in a position which makes them easy to access.

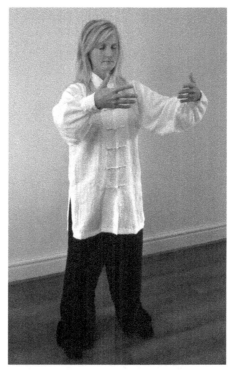

Figure 5.8: Zhan Zhuang

In this position your feet should be at shoulders' width apart, your spine upright and your head suspended. Ensure that you do not lean backwards as this will shut down important meridians which run through your back. I would like to reiterate this point now, do not lean backwards. This is of vital importance in your practice; most students who I teach at first lean backwards without realising that they are doing so. Even students who have come from outside schools, with years of prior experience, still lean backwards and it takes me quite a while to re-programme their posture to get them stood upright. Your shoulders should be relaxed and your arms held in front of you as if you are holding a ball. Do not have the hands too far from the body and ensure that they are not limp.

When first beginning this posture it is common for the arms and shoulders to have a great deal of pain and many students want to quit; don't give up. The pain is usually caused by excessive tension stored in your shoulders. Ask yourself if you need as much muscular force as you are using to hold your arms up; for most I am guessing that the answer is no. Beginners will only manage a few minutes before they have to relax their arms down and shake out the tension but with practice it does not take long before you are able to hold the posture for some time. I believe that everybody, within a few weeks of constant practice, should be able to get to around 45 minutes in this position very easily which is a perfect amount of time for this practice. If your Qi is flowing smoothly then the arms will seem to 'float' and there will be no pain. Several hours in this position will be easily manageable.

Now take your awareness and place it onto the Yuan source point of the Lung meridian: Taiyuan or Lung 9 (LU9) depending upon whether you prefer the names or the more modern numbering system. This is accomplished in exactly the same manner as when you placed your awareness into your palms in the previous exercise. Let your awareness connect to the Yuan source point on both wrists and let it rest there. Do not worry about anything else, just let your mind focus on the task and allow all outside concerns to fade away.

Over time you will get the same reaction as before, the Qi will start to be led down to the point due to the location of your awareness (Yi). At first it may wash up and down the arm but then it will reach the point where your mind is resting and the point will begin to activate. This is experienced as a sense of heat and pressure in the area. Some of my students have told me that it feels as though there is somebody gently squeezing the point as they carry out this part of the exercise.

Remember that Qi is a form of vibratory information. It is information which can be interpreted by the brain in numerous ways depending upon the quality of the information. This means that while everybody's experience of this stage will be similar there will still be variations. Do not worry if your brain interprets the activating of the Yuan source points in a slightly different way.

Remain here for some time, keep your awareness on this point, breathe deeply and continue to observe what is taking place. Perhaps this will be as far as you get in your first few attempts; if this is the case, don't worry about it. Everything takes practice and with time and perseverance you will progress.

After some time the Yi will begin to thread its way down into the meridian via the point. The Qi being led here by the breath serves as a translator between your mind and meridian and so the pathway of the meridian will open up for you. It is most likely that due to the depth of the meridian below the elbow it will only be this section of the meridian which appears at first. You will get a tangible sense of the pathway running from the elbow to the tip of the thumb as shown in Figure 5.9.

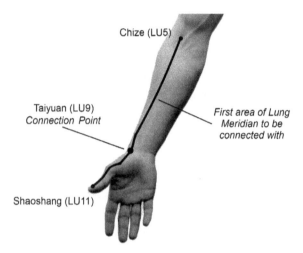

Figure 5.9: The Opening of the Lung Meridian

For a lot of people, this experience is quite a big step in their progress into the internal arts. I have had many students who were long time practitioners of Chinese medicine or Qi Gong. They had worked with Qi for a long time but never had a tangible experience of the meridian pathway like this before. It gives me the greatest pleasure to see them begin to smile as the meridian opens up for them and they begin to experience, for the first time, the nature of their own energy body. If you can achieve this then you are progressing in the correct direction and you are on the threshold of a whole internal landscape which can be explored with the mind.

The feeling of the meridian will vary from person to person and will largely depend upon the health of the meridian itself. We will discuss these feelings later in the book. Look for a sensation of pressure, heat or movement beneath the skin. Be aware though that this is not a subtle

ENTERING THE STREAM **125**

sensation. If you are unsure if it is real or if you have imagined it then put it down to your imagination; the sensation is so strong that it cannot be denied. You will not only be aware of the line of the meridian pathway but also the defined edges of the meridian giving it the feel of a thin three-dimensional tube which is running beneath the skin. Once the meridian has moved completely into the realm of sensation you will see that its pathway exactly matches the meridian charts passed down through the ages within Daoist medical practices; the same pathways reproduced in the previous chapter.

Stay with this practice for as long as you like. Enjoy the sensation of the Lung meridian. The only thing to note is that you should *not* try and *do* anything to the meridian. Just allow it to flow unimpeded by your mind and observe what is taking place. You may well become aware of a direction of flow through the meridian and it is a pleasant exercise just to observe this flow while you are standing there in Zhan Zhuang.

When you are ready to conclude your practice, lower your arms and walk briskly around the room for a few minutes.

The Arm Meridians

It is wise to begin connecting with the meridians of the arms first as they are far easier to feel than the leg meridians. From experience the following order seems to be the easiest:

- Lung meridian via Taiyuan (LU9)
- Large Intestine via Hegu (LI4)
- Pericardium via Daling (PC7)
- Triple Heater via Yangchi (TH4)
- Heart via Shenmen (HE7)
- Small Intestine via Wangu (SI4)

Connect with each meridian in the same way as for the Lung meridian. Follow the steps and progress gradually until you can get a tangible feeling of each meridian. Ensure that you can differentiate between the different meridians. It is likely that some meridians will be a great deal clearer than others; this is quite normal. Energy will have different qualities in different meridians and so your mind will find it easier to connect with some than others.

It is important not to over-think this part of the process. Follow the guidelines and just observe what is happening; with time your mind will become trained to locating the meridians of the arms and the process will become faster and easier. You are aiming to get to the stage where just a simple thought will produce the meridian for you. At this stage it is no longer necessary to use the Yuan source points, they have served their purpose for you as translators and are no longer needed. Yi alone will be enough.

Observations on the Arm Meridians

Here are some observations on the early stages of connecting with the meridians of the arm which have been drawn from my own and my students' experiences. Perhaps they will differ from your own observations but I have included them as they may be useful.

- The Lung meridian is generally the easiest to feel.

- The Large Intestine meridian tends to be much clearer on the hand than on the forearm at first. It quite often appears on the face below the nostril quite early as well although few people can feel the length of the meridian connecting the nostrils to the index finger when they are first starting out with this practice.

- The Pericardium meridian feels particularly strong around the area of Laogong (PC8) in the centre of the palm.

- The Heart is quite often a little painful for some people, a sharp aching sensation.

The Leg Meridians

The meridians which run to and from the feet tend to be more difficult to feel than the arms. This is likely due to the fact that our legs are usually carrying our weight so they tend to store more tension than the arms. Like the arms, the meridians of the leg tend to be closer to the surface nearer the extremities. From the knees to the feet they are much easier to feel with a couple of exceptions.

Follow the same process as for the arms when studying the meridians of the legs. Use the same Zhan Zhuang position as above at first but if this proves too difficult then try the exercise lying on your back. I personally found it much easier standing in Zhan Zhuang when I was learning but many of my students have reported the opposite. Find the position which works best for you.

The easiest order to follow when connecting with the leg meridians seems to be:

- Kidney via Yongquan (KI1), despite this not being the Yuan source point
- Spleen via Taibai (SP3)
- Liver via Taichong (LV3)
- Stomach via Chongyang (ST42)
- Bladder via Jingu (BL64)
- Gall Bladder via Qiuxu (GB40)

Note that it is easier to connect with the meridians via these points if they are uncovered so you may wish to take off your socks and shoes. However, the fact that your awareness and energy are coming together on these points will also mean that they are more susceptible to outside influences. If your practice area is cold or damp then this may cause blockages to enter the meridian during your practice; ensure that your practice space is warm and comfortable before beginning to connect with the meridians on the leg. Figure 5.10 shows the location of the main points on the leg through which you may connect with the meridians.

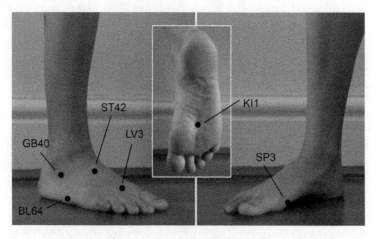

Figure 5.10: Leg Connection Points

The Kidney meridian is unique in that it does not utilise the Yuan source point as a point of entry for the mind. I have noted through practice and teaching these exercises that while the Yuan point of the Kidney meridian may be used it is actually easier through Yongquan (KI1). This is most likely due to the fact that this point's main function is to draw in energy from the planet. Since it is always drawing in information it lends itself towards drawing in the awareness.

Observations on the Leg Meridians

The following are some observations on the meridians of the legs, which have been drawn from my own and others' practice:

- The Kidney meridian tends to be quite uncomfortable-feeling for most people. This is due to the fact that many people overly burden their essence which drains the Kidneys. Contacting this meridian can be tiring and make you feel emotionally quite flat. If this happens do not worry, just work more on the other meridians until you have learnt how to rebalance the internal environment of your body as discussed later in the book.

- The Spleen meridian often appears on the ribs as well, near the conclusion of its external pathway.

- The Liver meridian can also come with a sensation of fullness in the groin area due to its pathway.

- The Bladder meridian can often be felt along the length of the spine quite early. It is a very quick meridian to feel in its entirety due to its shallow location in the body compared to the other meridians.

Continuing this Practice

It is wise to continue this practice for some time before moving on. Spend a few weeks at the least but ideally a few months practising these techniques daily. Ensure that you continue until you have a strong sense of the location of each of the meridians and that you can find them easily with just the use of your awareness. The better foundation you build here, the stronger your further practices will be.

If you have managed these stages well then you are beginning to move into the early stages of internal exploration of the meridian system. In the next chapter we will take this further and begin to analyse the nature of the meridians and how imbalance is felt within these Heavenly Streams of information.

CHAPTER 6

FURTHER EXPLORATION

The meridians not only serve to connect us to the powers of Heaven and Earth; they also transmit their information throughout the body. As Yin and Yang intermingle with each other to produce the six environmental energies they begin to have an effect upon the quality of the Qi that flows through us. If we are healthy and live our lives in synchronisation with the world we live within then this process will cause us no harm. The vast majority of people within modern society do not live in this way and health is generally pretty poor across the world. One result of this is that the energy of the environment often begins to move into the meridian system creating imbalance which begins to change the nature of our internal environment. This is the way in which disease from an external source takes a hold of us according to the Daoist medical tradition.

Disease from an internal source is usually generated from excessive emotional disturbance which begins to affect the related Zang Fu organ of the body, or from poor diet and lifestyle. Figure 6.1 summarises the process of imbalance developing from both internal and external sources.

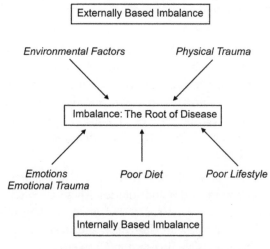

Figure 6.1: Internal and External Disease

This imbalance manifests in several ways within the body. These manifestations appear within the consciousness, energy body and physical body. With practice we can learn to find these signs and read them to discover the nature of our own imbalance. If we are able to identify the nature of our personal imbalance then we are also able to begin changing this imbalance.

The location and nature of imbalance within the three bodies of man:

- Within the consciousness imbalance will begin to disconnect us from the divine spiritual energy of Heaven and Dao. This is a very delicate connection and one that is quickly severed; from the second we are born our connection to the divine is constantly under attack from both internal and external sources. Manifestations of imbalances at this level are tendencies towards different emotional disturbances and psychological imbalances.

- Within the energy body there will be internal manifestations of the six environmental energies which will lead to blockages and disturbances within the meridians. This is covered in greater detail within this chapter.

- On a very deep level, the five elemental energies which circulate within the energetic cage of the congenital meridians will move out of balance. Since these energies lie at the core of a person's energetic being they will have a knock on effect on the rest of the body. It is for this reason that the Wu Xing Qi Gong were discussed early in the book and why they are recommended as practices to build a foundation for the exercises contained within the rest of this book.

- The energetic Zang Fu organ functions will begin to become disturbed either by the blockages which have appeared within the meridians from external sources or by energetic imbalances derived from internal sources. The signs of these energetic dysfunctions can be read as they manifest externally upon the physical body. These external manifestations are discussed in detail in Chapter 9.

- Within the physical body they can also manifest as various physical abnormalities and injuries. These are often overlooked as having an energetic source but understanding this is a large part of learning how to clear them and returning balance to the body. These are also discussed in Chapter 8.

The Energetic Connection

Whether these imbalances manifest within the consciousness body, the energy body or the physical body they are all connected to one another. A disease may manifest within the physical world, as in the case of trauma, but it will still affect the energy and consciousness body. In the same way, an imbalance within the mind will also manifest within both the energetic and physical bodies. This is a very useful fact for practitioners of the Daoist arts as it means that breaking the connection between the imbalances will cause them to begin to clear and good health can be restored. How do we break this connection? We work with the middle of the link: the energy body. This is the basis of the practices within this book and also within all Daoist medical practices such as acupuncture. In modern times there is an incorrect belief that ancient Chinese medical practitioners did not understand the physical body; this is not true. Although they understood the physical body, they realised that the most effective way to restore balance was to work directly with the energy body which would have a knock on effect to both the consciousness and the physical organs and tissues. Figure 6.2 summarises this concept.

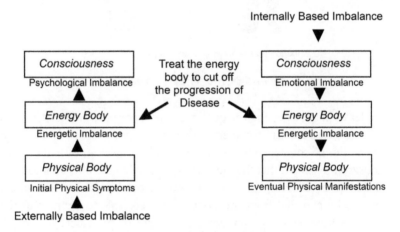

Figure 6.2: Energetic Imbalance

We have already learnt how to access this energy body in the previous chapter and by now you should be able to gain a strong connection to the meridians via the use of your Yi. If you have not yet achieved this level of ability then return to the previous practices until you can clearly feel the different meridian pathways. Please note that it can take a long time before you manage to feel the pathways of the meridians above the elbows and knees. These areas of the meridian system run much deeper within the body. Figure 6.3 shows the areas where the meridians are most easily connected to.

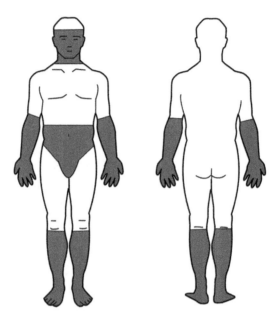

Shaded Areas = Areas of Easy Energetic Connection

Figure 6.3: Areas of Easy Connection

In order to begin assessing the quality of the energy within the meridians you need only be able to feel them within these areas of the body although you should, of course, continue towards feeling them all over the body. The reason for this is that the meridian system will naturally want to clear imbalances by moving them down towards the hands and feet where they can be expelled from the body. If you are able to connect to the meridians here then you can assess the nature of the blockages within each individual energetic pathway and with time learn how to assist in the clearing out process.

Meridian Qi Flow Quality

If you have been practising connecting with the meridians for some time then by now you will most likely have begun to note that the quality of the Qi flowing in each meridian is quite individual. Remember that the organs and their associated meridians are each linked to different elemental energies as well, meaning that the information contained within each meridian will vary as it flows through the body. It is these individual qualities that ensure that the Zang Fu organs and meridians are able to communicate with the physical body.

Unless a meridian has blockages present within it, it will have the following properties. These were taken from my own personal experience as well as the experience of the many students I have taught to connect with and assess their own (and others') meridians.

Heart and Small Intestine Meridians

The Qi flowing within the Heart and Small Intestine meridians is of the Fire element. It should feel expansive within the meridian, meaning that these meridians should feel wider than the other meridians of the arms. It is a warm feeling energy which flows quite slowly through the body with gentle pulses. Those in touch with their emotional state will often find that they begin to smile when they connect with these meridians; they can give a very comforting feeling.

Spleen and Stomach Meridians

This is Earth elemental energy. It moves with quite a high degree of force behind it and should give the feeling of information being pushed through the meridians. Within the Spleen meridian (but not so much within the Stomach meridian) you should be able to feel it surging up through the body, especially around the feet and the meridian point of Gongsun (SP4). Those who manage to connect their emotional state successfully with this meridian will begin to feel very calm, the mind will move into a still state and many of my students have described it as feeling as though they are 'mesmerised' by the pulsing of the Spleen meridian.

Lungs and Large Intestine Meridians

The energy flowing through the Lung and Large Intestine meridians is of the Metal element. It is a contracting energy which pulls in towards the centre which means that these meridians can feel quite tight. When the lines of these meridians appear it is as if they are tightly bound and for many people feel far less pleasant than the other meridians. The movement of Qi within these meridians tends to be quite subtle resulting in it often seeming as though the Qi is standing still (though this is not the case). It is also common for people to feel that the meridian is quite cold; an almost 'menthol' like sensation.

Kidney and Bladder Meridians

The Kidney and Bladder meridians contain Water elemental energy. This energy feels as if it runs like fluid through the body. It is easy to understand how the elemental energies gained their names as after a while it does feel distinctly as if there is water running through the body through the pathways of the Kidney and Bladder meridians; remember that the elemental energies gained their names from inner examination of their nature. It is a fast moving energy which feels as if it flows down the back of the body and shoots up through the legs through the Kidney meridians. It is interesting that the meridian point name Yongquan (KI1) means 'Bubbling Spring' and is an indication of the feeling which can be experienced at this point. It is much like you are stood in a Jacuzzi and bubbles are being pushed up below your foot. This meridian point name hails back to the times when the meridians were still studied experientially as opposed to through the intellectual methods of learning institutions today.

Liver and Gall Bladder Meridians

The Wood elemental energy of the Liver and Gall Bladder meridians is the fastest moving and most forceful of the meridian energies. It forces its way through the meridians and the direction of flow can easily be felt within these meridians. Wood elemental energy is slightly warm but not as warm as the Fire elemental energy of the Heart and Small Intestine meridians. It is common for those who have just finished a session of connecting with the Wood elemental meridians to feel very 'driven' afterwards. For a short time afterwards they often feel energised.

Pericardium and Triple Heater Meridians

Although the Qi within the Pericardium and Triple Heater meridians is warm and expansive as with the Heart and Small Intestine meridians it has one distinct qualitative difference: it moves very slowly. It feels very thick and has been compared by my students to a flow of honey running through their meridians. Perhaps this is one of the reasons that the Pericardium and Triple Heater meridians are often separated from the other Fire elemental meridians? This Qi has a very smooth flowing feel; the surge of the other Fire elemental meridians is experienced as a much more subtle and slow force.

Individuality of Experience

Since Qi is only a vibrational form of information which is translated by the mind, it can be interpreted in many ways. The way in which your own brain reads the information contained within the Qi you are connecting with may vary slightly from the information contained within this chapter. This is not a problem although your experience will likely be something very similar to this. Your brain will interpret the information as something you can understand and process; according to the Daoist tradition this is the same process which converts Qi to 'trick' you into thinking that the physical world is real. What you will realise though is that your meridians are definitely not just an ancient misunderstanding of nerves, lymph and other physical aspects of the body as is taught within many contemporary schools of Chinese medicine and Qi Gong. They are a network of energetic information quite different from any part of the physical systems studied within Western medical science.

Studying the Meridians

When you are getting a feel for the quality of the different meridians you should connect with them as before and then begin to run your awareness up and down their length. Simply move your mind up and down very gently so that you do not change the nature of the Qi running through each energetic pathway. Keep your focus gentle and relaxed, do not picture anything, instead simply explore. As before, you should 'listen' to what the meridian is saying and gradually the different qualities of the Qi flowing here will begin to unfold and present themselves to you.

The above description of the meridians applies if the energy here is balanced and healthy. These sensations will vary if there are any blockages or imbalances present along their length. Please note that you should never worry if you do find imbalances; it is quite normal. I would argue that nobody should find all of their meridians to be perfectly healthy and clear. If you do find this to be the case then I would suggest that you continue to explore them; with time you should find that this is not the case.

Each of the environmental energies discussed in Chapter 4 may manifest within the meridians along with general stagnation, deficiency of Qi and Phlegm which is a by-product of the body due to the presence of stagnation. Each of these imbalances has their own energetic imprint, their own vibrational frequency. These imprints can be found within the meridian system as you run your awareness along the length of the meridians; these imprints will each produce their own sensations which are discussed below.

- *Wind Heat:* This is an easily changeable energy which moves through the length of the meridians. Its location is difficult to pin down as it is constantly shifting. Generally any blockage that feels as if it is moving is related to the energy of Wind. This pathogen will also be felt as an area of uncomfortable heat sat within the meridian.

- *Wind Cold:* Like Wind Heat, this pathogen moves through the meridian making its exact location difficult to pin down. The sensation is of an uncomfortably cold area within the pathway of the meridian.

- *Cold:* Cold pathogenic information is very unpleasant to connect with. It is felt as a dull ache which is localised to the area of the meridian within which the Cold is sitting. It is particularly common within the joints of the body. It always feels cold. In extreme cases it can feel almost as if there were ice sat in the meridian.

- *Damp:* Damp blocks the meridians, leading to deficiency of energy flow in that area of the body. It is a heavy feeling pathogen that feels as if the meridian has swollen to accommodate the pathogen. It can feel as if the area of the body where the meridian is running has become swollen once your awareness connects with this pathogen.

- *Dryness:* Dryness in the meridian feels sticky. It is as if the Qi flowing through this area of the meridian has a slightly rough and adhesive quality. It is often accompanied by a feeling of warmth. This is the least common imbalance to come into contact with within the meridians.

- *Heat:* When your awareness connects with this pathogen it is common to feel a heat in the meridian which can vary from uncomfortable to almost burning. It is always a localised pathogen which will aim to reach the extremities ready for clearing;

consequently it is fairly easy to clear although if the body is in a state of producing internal Heat then more will follow.

- *Stagnant Qi:* This feels like an uncomfortable pressure in the meridian. It is a difficult sensation to pin down but can be compared to the feeling you have when pressing on a bruise. This is one of the most common imbalances to feel within the length of the meridian.

- *Qi Deficiency:* Connecting with a meridian which is deficient of Qi is like finding an empty tube. Unlike many of the other imbalances listed here, Qi deficiency tends to be felt in the quality of the entire meridian rather than being localised to one point.

- *Qi Excess:* Excessive Qi will result in a feeling of the energy within that meridian being overwhelming. The Qi surges with a pulse that can be felt by the awareness. It is much like the entire meridian has its own heart-beat.

- *Phlegm:* Phlegm within the meridian refers to an energetic imprint which can also manifest as the physical substance of phlegm when it reaches the organs of the body. Within the meridians it is still in an energetic state. When the awareness connects with Phlegm in the meridian it is as if there is a hard nodule within the length of the meridian. This is a strong blockage which has a very tangible sensation to it.

- *Blood Stasis:* If Qi stagnates within a meridian it can also lead to Blood Stasis within that area of the body. This will be felt as a sharp pain which only becomes apparent when the awareness passes along this area of the meridian.

These are key imbalances which may manifest within the length of the meridians. In many cases you may not be able to differentiate between certain types of imbalance; some of them are quite similar in feeling when you first begin this practice. Do not worry too much, in many cases the meridians can simply be dredged (as discussed later) which will serve to free up most imbalances from the length of the channels. With time you will be able to differentiate between the different imbalances with ease. Figure 6.4 summarises the various qualities of these energetic imbalances.

Wind Heat
Wind Cold

A moving imbalance which is often
accompanied by either a sensation of
hot or cold

Cold

A dull ache localised within the Meridian
Pathway. Often located in the area of the
body's joints. Cold feeling

Damp

A feeling of swelling within the Meridian.
Often accompanied by a feeling of
heaviness or sinking

Dryness

The Qi flowing here has a rough or slightly
adhesive quality as though it is sticking

Heat

A feeling of heat or burning. In extreme
cases it can feel as though there is a
fire within the Meridian Pathway

Stagnant Qi

A feeling of pressure in the Meridian.
Similar to pressing on a bruise

Qi Deficient

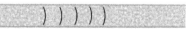

A feeling of emptiness within the length
of the Meridian. Not normally localised
to one area

Qi Excess

A feeling of a surging force along the
meridian. It is as if the Meridian has
a very distinctive pulse

Phlegm

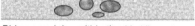

Phlegm nodules within the Meridian are
very clear blockages to feel

Figure 6.4: Energetic Imbalances

Exploring the Three Heaters

As well as assessing the length of the meridians for imbalances it is also wise to assess the quality of the Qi within the three energetic chambers of the Triple Heater. These three areas of the energy body which are linked to the functioning of the three Dan Tien are vitally important for the distribution of Jing, Qi, Shen and body fluids through the body. If there is a weakness in one of the chambers of the Triple Heater it is common for there to be imbalance within the organs and tissues local to that area.

To assess the health of the Triple Heater we need to connect with the Qi within that area so that our awareness can begin to take a reading of the level of balance there. When connecting with the Triple Heater we move from bottom to top. Figure 6.5 shows the three energetic chambers of the Triple Heater.

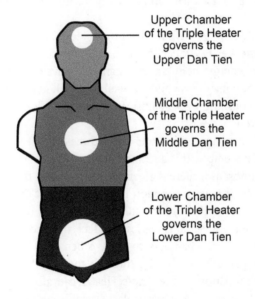

Figure 6.5: The Triple Heater

Please note that this is an understanding of the Triple Heater according to the Daoist tradition drawn from internal practices rather than the understanding according to contemporary Chinese medical practices.

Stand in the Zhan Zhuang position used during your earlier practice of connecting with the individual meridians. Now bring your mind in to the lower chamber of the Triple Heater. Rather than focusing on a specific point or meridians, you should expand your awareness to fill the whole area shown in Figure 6.5. Allow the resulting sensation to give you an understanding of the nature of the Qi within this area of the energy system. Now repeat this process for the middle and upper energetic chambers of the Triple Heater.

It is very difficult to feel the health of the three chambers of the Triple Heater individually. They must be compared to each other to ascertain how they feel. This is because the nature of the three chambers relate to each other very closely; theirs is a relationship of balance, flow and equalisation. Imbalance within the Triple Heater will manifest as an uneven amount of energy across the three chambers. It is most common for one of the three chambers to stand out from the other two as being of a different quality; usually we understand these qualities in terms of being too excessive or too weak. At an early stage of Triple Heater imbalance this will manifest in the ways described below but with time it will begin to manifest as imbalance within the organs that reside within this area of the body.

Excessive energy within one of the three chambers will feel as though the Qi in the area is swollen. Note that this is a sensation of being swollen within the energy body rather than the physical body although the physical body may be swollen as well. You will get a sense of the energy in this area pushing back against your awareness; it will usually feel quite heavy as well.

Deficient energy within one of the three chambers feels as if that area of the body is empty. It is a strange sensation but one that it very clear to feel. It is almost as if there is an empty space within that whole area of the energy body. It is very common for people to get this sensation around the middle Heater if they have suffered some kind of emotional trauma.

As stated above, it is easiest to feel these differences when you compare the three chambers to each other. This will give you a feel of the comparative flow of Qi through the length of the entire Triple Heater. Examination of the Triple Heater can also help to give you an understanding of why a particular organ is weak. For example, you may have a tendency towards a weakness of energy within the Lungs and Heart. Upon examination of the energy of the Triple Heater it is discovered that the middle Heater is deficient in energy. Rebalancing this issue may rely not only on nourishing the energy of the Lungs and Heart but also the middle energetic chamber of the Triple Heater.

Exploring External Manifestations

So far we have looked at the theory of the energy system and in particular the meridians. We have looked at how to connect with and assess the energy body to look for imbalances. This will, with practice, give us insight into the nature of our own imbalances but we also have one other method of understanding our energetic health. This method is the observation of external signs. External signs of imbalance are physical symptoms which are similar to those which are observed by Western doctors at the observational stage of developing a diagnosis. For example, a cough is a clear sign of imbalance within the Lungs. Although this example is fairly obvious, some of the other signs are not so clearly linked to the organs when you first begin to study them. Through developing an understanding of the nature of organs according to Daoism, though, it is possible to see why these signs indicate various imbalances.

In the next chapter the various energetic functions of the Zang (Yin) and Fu (Yang) organs of the body are discussed. These functions then have a strong connection to the physical realm as Qi changes to Jing and forms matter. Understanding the nature of the Zang Fu organ energetic functions builds a strong foundation upon which to understand the external signs of imbalance which are covered in Chapter 8. With all of this information it is then possible to gain a clear understanding of the nature of your own imbalance and then to form a strategy for dealing with this imbalance.

CHAPTER 7

THE EARTHLY FRUIT

This chapter looks at the Yin and Yang organs of the body as well as the extra Fu organs. This is an understanding of physiology according to the Daoist tradition which is important foundational knowledge for any practitioners of the internal arts. Those who are not already familiar with the nature of the human body according to Daoism should study this chapter closely before proceeding onto the exercises in the later sections of this book.

The Daoist view of the human body and its organs differs greatly from the Western scientific understanding. Modern medicine has clearly defined physical functions for each of the body's organs. These are functions which can clearly be observed and measured within the physical realm. The Daoist view is quite different from this; just as with everything else in the universe the Daoists divide the nature of the human bodily organs into three broad categories: their spiritual attributes, their energetic functions and finally their physical manifestation. If we look at the organs in this way then they suddenly take on very different roles from their Western scientific counterparts.

Spiritual Attributes of the Organs

Each of the organs of the body has a link to human consciousness and spirituality. The foundation of the physical world lies within the realm of pure consciousness and the bodily organs are no different. Disturbances within any organ of the body will have a knock on effect within the mind and vice versa. The primary organs even house various aspects of the human spirit, and understanding these enables us to understand the undeniable connection which exists between mind and body. The spiritual aspects of the organs are governed by Shen.

BOX 7.1: NON-DEFINITION OF DISEASE

The Daoist understanding of disease is very different from the modern Western concept of sickness which the majority of us will have grown up with. Modern Western style doctors work by looking at the various symptoms we have, carrying out a variety of tests and then giving us a final diagnosis. This sickness or condition is defined by its nature and, in essence, its similarity to cases which have been seen in the past.

The Daoist understanding of sickness is different. There is no defined diagnosis; instead their medicine is based upon looking to understand the nature of what is taking place within the environment of the body at that particular time. Which organ is currently energetically out of balance? Where is the blockage present within the Jing Luo system and how is the body reacting to the external world? The resulting reading of energetic imbalance may shift and change as time goes on. Indeed an illness that we understand as being asthma, for example, may be down to a deficiency of Lung Qi, a weakness of the Kidneys' energy or an imbalance within the energy of the Spleen as well as due to emotional disturbances or environmental energies invading the body. Over time these conditions will change as nothing is constant within Daoism.

The key difference between these two approaches is that within Daoism nothing is defined in a concrete manner. Modern medicine seeks to define and label a disease while the Daoist approach is simply to understand the nature of the energy body right now. Why is this? The answer is simple. Once something is defined it is much more difficult to change. The Daoism approach enables us to work with a shifting energy to effectively bring about change to a situation. This lack of definition is of key importance when trying to improve health through a Daoist medicinal practice. Sadly, many contemporary Chinese medicine practitioners do not understand this and so concrete definition of disease has crept into their practice. It is common for an acupuncturist to try and treat you for asthma when they should instead be staying true to the ancient way of understanding sickness.

Does this mean you should ignore your Western diagnosis? No, definitely not. Western medicine has saved countless lives and is very advanced. Instead I am saying that you should step back from the diagnosis when trying to work in the way outlined within this book. If you have asthma and you rely on Western inhalers then obviously do not stop taking them; but when you are sitting down to practise the point activation from this book you should temporarily try to put that diagnosis to the back of your mind. Try to forget the label which is difficult to change. Just try to understand the nature of the energy within you as outlined in this book then go through the process to try and change that energy. If energy is truly fluid and non-defined then it is far more likely to change.

Energetic Functions of the Human Body

As the frequency of spiritual energy begins to lessen it moves into the energetic realm; the realm of Qi. It is within this range of frequencies that the energetic functions of the human bodily organs exist. It is also from here that the meridian system stretches out to connect our consciousness with our physical body; an intermediary that enables life to form between Heaven and Earth. Each of these energetic functions is a reflection of the movements taking place within the spiritual aspect of each organ and it is these functions which usually cause the most confusion to anybody comparing modern physiology to Daoist teachings.

Physical Manifestations

When the Qi begins to condense down into the next realm of existence, the physical form is brought into existence. Here the physical organ comes into existence. Seen as the leaves on a tree rather than the root, the physical organs owe their existence to the energy body and prior to this pure consciousness. It is here, within the physical realm, that modern Western medicine places 100 per cent of its focus when studying the bodily organs and here that, arguably, the Daoists placed least importance. To the Daoists, the majority of sicknesses within the physical body could be traced back to energetic disturbances and prior to that the mind.

The Zang and the Fu

The organs of the body are divided into two broad categories: Yin organs which are known as the Zang organs and the Yang organs which are known as the Fu organs. The Yin (Zang) organs are seen as the governing organs and the most important with regards to their functions. They are usually understood to be more solid than the Yang organs and closely linked to the process of making, storing and regulating the various substances of the body. The Yang (Fu) organs are seen as hollow organs which deal mostly with receiving, distributing and finally excreting substances within the body. Each Yin organ is linked to a Yang organ and these two work as a pair, supporting each other in various ways. The paired Yin and Yang organs are summarised in Table 7.1.

Table 7.1: The Zang and Fu Organs

Yin (Zang) Organs	Yang (Fu) Organs
Heart	Small Intestine
Spleen	Stomach
Lungs	Large Intestine
Kidneys	Bladder
Liver	Gall Bladder
Pericardium	Triple Heater

The studies of Nei Gong, Qi Gong and indeed any of the other internal arts including meditation are one method of study of our own inner universe. The Daoist practices are a study of what takes place on each of the three levels: the spiritual, the energetic and the physical. It is useful for us to have an understanding of the functions and relationships of the Yin and Yang organs of the body. Remember that everything within the universe is reflected on multiple levels. That which takes place within us also takes place within the macrocosm of the environment we live within. A deep understanding of our own inner universe can lead to a high level of understanding of the movements of energy within the outside world. This was one of the original tenets of Daoism.

It is important that you keep in mind the threefold nature of organ functions according to Daoism as you read the next section of the book. Here each organ is discussed in detail according to its ancient understanding. Remember that when the word Heart appears, for example, it refers to the Heart on a spiritual, energetic and physical level; not just the physical organ. If you can adjust your mind so that it always sees the organs in this way, it will help you in your understanding of Daoism.

The Yin (Zang) Organs
The Heart (Xin)
The Heart is born of pure Fire consciousness or energy. The spiritual light of Fire is the expanding, warming light of comprehension. It gives us the aspect of consciousness known as spirit (Shen). The Heart also governs the movement of Blood (Xue) through the body which provides nourishment to the rest of the organs and tissues.

Spiritual Attributes

Our Spirit (Shen) is that which connects us to the divine. It is the power of enlightenment, intuition and understanding. The Shen aspect of consciousness has the highest frequency vibration and is the most refined manifestation of the energy which moves through us. Shen provides us with a link to the divine powers of Heaven and Dao as long as we know how to nurture and communicate with our own innate wisdom. This is the spiritual function of the Heart; it is a storehouse for the Shen.

It is interesting to note that the Chinese character for Heart shows an empty hollow rather than an organ. This is the profound truth of the Heart, in order for it to remain healthy it relies on being empty. Our spirit resides within the empty space at the centre of our consciousness. Here it lays and carries out its role of connecting us to Heaven but if disturbances cause the emptiness to fill then the spirit is disturbed and communication can no longer take place. What is it that fills this empty space and disturbs the spirit? It is our emotions. Emotions are energetic disturbances of the mind which prevent us from connecting to our own spirit. Any strong emotional disturbance has a negative effect upon the Heart. This is why Daoism always places a great emphasis on quieting the emotions and connecting with the emptiness. They refer to this process as 'stilling the Heart'.

Energetic Functions

When the spiritual light of Fire reaches the energetic realm, the result is Fire Qi. The Fire Qi circulates through the body via the meridians linked to this element including the Heart meridian. This energy also governs the various energetic functions linked to the Heart. At this stage though, nothing is physically manifested. This is the realm of Qi and function, of information, not matter and form.

The Yang function of the Heart is the propulsion of Blood through the body. Blood is one of the vital substances of the human body. Figure 7.1 shows the functions of Blood (Xue).

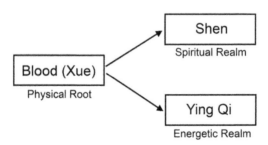

Figure 7.1: The Functions of Blood

Consciousness is the root of all creation but physicality is the anchor of energy and consciousness. Each relies on the other for existence. The Daoist view of Blood is that it is the physical anchor and vehicle for Ying Qi and Shen.

Ying Qi is the form of energy which travels throughout the body and keeps it functioning. It is the information which keeps the whole energy body alive. Without Ying Qi everything would cease to function on an energetic level which would in turn cause the physical body to die. The Ying Qi travels with the blood which is propelled by the Heart.

As we have seen already, Shen sits within the emptiness at the centre of the Heart. From here some of it moves through the body via the blood. This enables human consciousness to communicate with the rest of the body which means that the health of our Shen has a direct influence on the health of our organs on a physical level.

The Yin function of the Heart is to help in the creation of the Ying Qi. It puts this energy into the Blood along with the Shen which is delivered throughout the body.

Physical Manifestations

The Fire energy when it reaches the physical realm creates the physical organ of the heart as we understand it in Western science. It also manifests in the tongue and the facial complexion.

Figure 7.2 gives an overview of the various functions of the Heart.

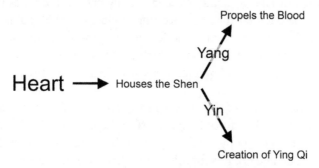

Figure 7.2: The Various Functions of the Heart

The Spleen (Pi)

The dividing energy of the spiritual light of Earth gives us our intellect, awareness and focus; the aspect of our consciousness known as Yi. It also governs our body's ability to transform and transport various substances within the body via the movements of the Spleen.

Spiritual Attributes

Our Yi is the ability of our mind to focus on tasks. Within Daoism, the Yi listens to the spiritual lessons of the Shen, which is in turn communicating with Heaven and the Dao. This means that it enables us to convert our divine inspiration into directed intentions and actions. This is the transformative power of the spirit which dictates the various functions of the Spleen.

According to Daoism we are essentially spiritual beings who should act on the messages given to us by the Shen. This is known as 'following the mandate of Heaven' and has always been the ideal way of Daoism. If the Yi is not able to carry out this communication then the Earth energy can become disturbed which leads to worry and an obsession with trivial concerns. The spleen is the physical manifestation of this aspect of our consciousness and it is particularly easy to damage through poor diet. This means that eating unhealthily will unbalance the Yi and lead to an inability to focus and communicate with our Shen.

Energetic Functions

The Yang energetic function of the Spleen is to hold up the other organs of the body. Each of the five elemental energies have a specific way of moving. The energy of Earth which governs the Spleen divides before evolving into a new energy. This is the energy of division and transformation. The dividing manifestation of the Earth energy within the Spleen dictates its ability to send healthy energy and fluids upwards through the body for further processing while the 'turbid' fluids are sent downwards to the large intestine for further processing and separation. It is the energy moving upwards which holds everything in place. If this aspect of the Spleen has become weakened then the organs are prone to prolapse.

The Yang aspect of the Spleen also governs the ability to absorb the Qi from our food and drink and transform it into an energy which we may use within the body. This energy absorbed from the food is the basis for our Blood and Qi. It is for this reason that the Spleen is often referred to as the root of our acquired energy.

The Yin energetic function of the Spleen is to help keep the Blood (Xue) within the blood vessels. If the Yin aspect becomes weak then it is possible that the Blood will escape the vessels resulting in a person being easily bruised. In extreme cases this may result in internal haemorrhaging.

Physical Manifestations

The physical manifestation of the Earth energy is the spleen as we understand it within Western biological sciences. It also manifests within the muscles of the body and the lips.

Figure 7.3 summarises the functions of the Spleen.

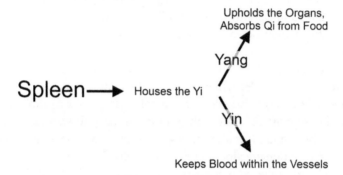

Figure 7.3: The Various Functions of the Spleen

The Lungs (Fei)

The spiritual light of Metal has a gently contracting directional force. It gives us the more physical aspect of our soul known as the Po. It also governs our ability to breathe and draw in Heavenly Qi as well as disperse fluids throughout the body via the actions of the Lungs.

Spiritual Attributes

The soul has two aspects to it within Daoism. The Yin aspect is our Po which connects us to the physical realm. It is the energy of sensory awareness and physical sensation. Without the Po we would have no connection to the world we live within and no ability to derive sensation from the experiences we have; sensory or emotional. A disturbance here can lead to a sensation of numbness, either physical or emotional. Emotionally the Lungs are linked to grief and sadness which are usually seen as emotions which are derived from some outside factor. This is the effect of the world on the Po; depending upon the state of the Po it may cause a person to react to difficult life events with varying degrees of sadness or numbness. It is no coincidence that the Lungs are also linked to the skin through which we feel physical sensation via the nervous system which is also usually linked to the Po.

It is said that inhalation and exhalation are reflections of the movements of the Po. Stress, sadness and difficulty disturb the Po which is a sensitive element of our consciousness. This in turn disturbs the breathing which has a knock on effect to the health of the rest of the body. Within ancient Daoist texts the Po was personified and seen as either one or sometimes seven fragile and emotional ghosts. These were acutely aware of their own mortality which caused them to become grief stricken reflecting the emotion of the Lungs. It is through breathing exercises that ancient Daoists aimed to calm the emotional Po which resided within the Lungs so that they would not cause disturbances which may in turn affect the Shen.

Disturbances within the Po are also linked to addictive behaviour. An overly dominant Po will seek physical stimulation in the form of an addiction. Whatever this addiction may be: drugs, sex, gambling or so forth, the Po must be dealt with in order to move forward and end the addictive behaviour. It is also interesting to note that the Po is said to be in charge of rational action and knowing what is healthy behaviour for the mind and body; weaknesses in the Po often lead to self-destructive behavioural patterns.

Energetic Functions

The Yang function of the Lungs is to draw in Heavenly Qi through our breathing. This energy moves through the body nourishing the organs, calming the mind and balancing the energy of the planet which we draw into the body through Yongquan. This energy which is drawn into the body combines with the energy drawn from our food by the actions of the Spleen. It is from a combination of these two types of energy that the various forms of acquired Qi within the body are drawn. This energy also governs the health of the two main Heavenly organs: the Heart and the Lungs.

The Lungs also help to expel pathogenic factors from the body. As we exhale, stagnant energy is removed from the body along with carbon dioxide via the movement of the physical lungs. A weakness in the Lungs will have a knock on effect to our ability to remove these pathogens and so internal sickness will develop.

The Yin function of the Lungs is to govern the dispersal of body fluids. The Lungs are compared to a canopy upon which the fluids of the body cool and condense. This fluid is then distributed back into the body, cooling and lubricating everything. These fluids keep the organs of the body, including the lungs, moist and if this function is compromised then the body can dry up. Along with these fluids is transported the body's sweat. If the Lungs are not working well then there can be irregularities with regards to how much a person sweats.

Physical Manifestations

The physical manifestations of the Metal energy are the lungs. This energy also manifests upon the skin, the body hair and within the nose.

Figure 7.4 summarises the various functions of the Lungs.

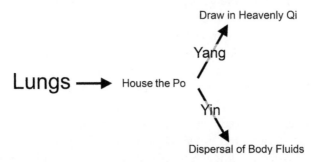

Figure 7.4: The Various Functions of the Lungs

The Kidneys (Shen)

Please note that although the Kidneys are called Shen in Chinese, this is different to the Shen of spirit. It uses a different tonal pronunciation and a different character. In order to avoid confusion the Kidneys will not be referred to in Chinese again within this book.

The sinking spiritual light of Water manifests as the mysterious aspect of our consciousness we know as Zhi, will-power. It also governs the motive energies of life and the body via the actions of the Kidneys.

Spiritual Attributes

The Kidneys are said to house the Zhi. This is often translated as meaning our will-power but, as with all things within Daoism, there is another layer to the meaning of Zhi. On a personal level our Zhi gives us the drive to get things done. It moves us forward in life with determination and grit in the face of difficulty. In an ideal, balanced state of consciousness it would be our Shen which gave us divine connection to the energy of Heaven above us, our Yi would convert these messages into conscious awareness and then our Zhi would give us the drive to see the resultant plans through. Alongside this is the Zhi of Dao. This is the will-power of the cosmos; the nearest translation to this may be 'destiny' although this word does not fit 100 per cent with the Daoist concept. In order to understand this concept we must first understand the concept of Ming. Ming is our 'pre-destined journey from life to death'. Physical death is an inevitability for everyone; how we get to this point will vary depending upon how we live. A person with a healthy connection to their Ming will move smoothly from point A to point B, birth to death, fulfilling various life goals and spiritually evolving. Longevity and good health will be theirs to enjoy; this is the ultimate path of Dao. It is the Zhi or 'will' of Heaven that everybody have this opportunity according to Daoist teachings. However, it is our actions which dictate whether or not we realise the Zhi of Heaven. Those who don't will have a rocky road ahead of them, and life is likely to be cut short by disease or calamity.

It is interesting to note here that the concept of Heaven's Zhi, the will of Heaven, is similar to the concept of Karma that many people are more familiar with but with a few differences. Rather than a form of cause and effect whereby one only affects one's own life the Daoist view is that our actions affect everybody around us due to the interconnected nature of existence. Although people all fall under the will of Heaven, we also, unfortunately, fall under the effects of each other. A person may be following the ideal path but sadly another's actions may negatively impact upon them. This can happen within the microcosm of one person's life but also on the macrocosm of world affairs. An example of this would be the starvation of people on a mass scale in parts of Africa; this would be seen within Daoist thought as a knock on effect of the actions of people in the Western world. Everything is connected; a great imbalance on one side of the world will create effects on the other.

Energetic Functions

The link between our Zhi, the Zhi of Heaven and our Ming is closely linked to the Yang energetic function of the Kidneys: the Ming Fire.

The Ming Fire is an energetic storehouse of information which governs the myriad functions of the human energetic system. Like a fire it creates an expansive, warming movement which radiates from the area of the kidneys out to the rest of the body. There is an acupuncture point on the governing meridian known as Mingmen (Gateway to our Ming) or GV4 which enables us to directly access this point and affect the Ming Fire.

The Ming Fire is a catalyst for the conversion of all acquired energy of the body from our original essence; our Jing. The Jing is the blueprint of the body, the seed for physical existence and the lowest frequency vibration of the three treasures of man: Jing, Qi and Shen. Our Jing moves downwards from the area of the kidneys to be transformed primarily into sexual fluid although it is also involved in the creation of Wei Qi; a form of vibrational energy which governs our ability to fight off externally originated disease. While some of the Jing is heading here, some of it travels into the lower Dan Tien to be converted into Qi which is then transported throughout the body along with the energies we breathe in and take from our food. In order for this to take place we need a motivating power and this is the Ming Fire. Like the spark which ignites a gas heating system, the Ming Fire enables the transformation of essence to take place. This is turn ensures that the body receives what it needs so that it can function efficiently.

The final job of the Ming Fire is to warm the organs of the body which do not like a cold environment, primarily these are the Spleen and the Stomach as well as the lower portion of the Triple Heater and the Bladder. If the Ming Fire is not burning strongly enough then these organs will not be adequately warmed and so they will not function properly.

Figure 7.5 summarises the functions of the Ming Fire.

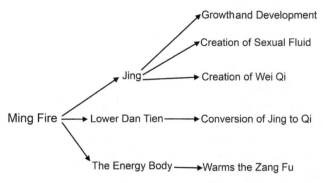

Figure 7.5: The Functions of the Ming Fire

The Yin energetic function of the Kidneys varies according to age. In children it governs growth and physical development. The Jing is used up as the child grows and matures. In adults this process changes and instead the Kidney's Yin energetic function relates to our sexuality and reproduction. The conversion of Jing to sexual fluids is happening constantly and it is because of this that excessive sex will deplete the Kidneys' Yin aspect.

The Kidneys also have two main functions which are not divided by Yin and Yang; they are quite unique in this way. First, they anchor the Lungs' energy which means that they assist in the Lungs' drawing in of Heaven Qi. If this anchor becomes weak then the Lungs can become negatively affected. Second they control the health of the Bones and the Brain. This is not actually a Kidney function but a function of the Jing. Since the Jing is controlled by the Kidneys then this function is usually assigned to the Kidneys themselves.

Physical Manifestations

The Water energy manifests as the kidneys, as they are usually understood within Western biological sciences, as it reaches the frequency of the physical realm. It also manifests in the health of the ears and the head hair.

Figure 7.6 summarises the various functions of the Kidneys.

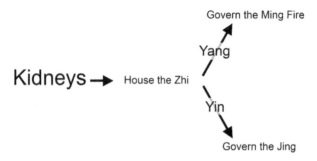

Figure 7.6: The Functions of the Kidneys

The Liver (Gan)

The spiritual light of Wood is fast moving and direct. It manifests within the human consciousness as the Yang aspect of our soul, the Hun. As it condenses into the energetic and then the physical realm it governs the movement of our Qi and the volume of our blood through the actions of the Liver.

Spiritual Attributes

The Yang or ethereal aspect of our soul is known as the Hun. This is the side of our consciousness that deals with imagination, dreams and planning. At night the Hun is said to reside within the Liver where it is rooted in the Liver Blood while at day the Hun is said to look out through our eyes. In these respects it is clear to see that it shares some properties with the Shen which is also rooted in Blood, although not specifically the Blood of the Liver, and can also be observed to connect with the eyes. The link between these two has to do with their more ethereal nature in comparison to the other aspects of our consciousness. The Shen and the Hun are said to be like clouds floating freely through the mind, connecting with the realms of Heaven and Dao while the Po and the Zhi have denser, more tangible connections to the realms of Jing and matter. Sat between these two poles is the Yi, the earthy, grounding aspect of thought, awareness and focus which serves as a pivot for the rest of the consciousness; a balance between Yin and Yang.

The Hun takes the insights given by the light of Shen and converts them into tangible plans. These plans are weighed up and affected by our dreams and aspirations. From here the Yi is able to observe the plans made by the Hun and turn these into thought and actions which are seen through via the driving force of the Zhi. Throughout this process the Po is present to provide rationale and sensory feedback.

Figure 7.7 summarises the interactions of the five spiritual aspects of human consciousness.

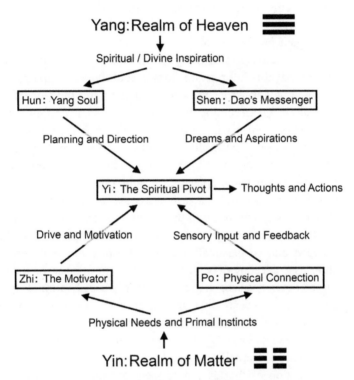

Figure 7.7: Interactions of the Five Spirits

The Hun is a wandering aspect of consciousness. It comes and goes freely resulting in dreams at night. Any major disturbances in the Hun are quickly manifested within the dreams. Because of the Hun's close relationship and communication with the Shen it became a part of Daoism to study a person's dreams to look for messages sent straight from Heaven. Since the language of the Hun is often symbolic rather than literal the study of dream analysis became a large part of the Daoist tradition. Prophetic dreams and suchlike are the result of gaining a strong connection with a healthy and balanced Hun.

The Hun is the planner. The weighing up of options and outcomes is the duty of the Hun along with the search for a life-path which will fulfil personal dreams and aspirations. The Zhi governs the will of Heaven and the Shen carries the messages of Heaven while the Hun governs a person's personal aspirations.

Energetic Functions

The Yang function of the Liver is to govern the smooth flow of Qi throughout the body. Qi in different parts of the body moves in different directions. The information superhighway of the energy body carries vibrational frequencies throughout all of the meridians and collaterals which connect consciousness to the physical body. It is the role of the Liver to ensure that this information flows smoothly and in the correct direction. A weakness in either the energy or the Yang function of the Liver will result in Qi becoming blocked and stagnant or flowing in the wrong direction, which will have adverse effects on the functioning of the body as a whole. The healthy directions of Qi according to the governance of the Liver are as follows: Lung, Stomach and Intestinal Qi should flow downwards while Spleen Qi should ascend. The directional flow of the other organs is not primarily governed by the Liver.

If Qi becomes stagnant through the function of the Liver becoming compromised then emotional frustration will begin to appear. The Hun will feel trapped and so personal dreams and aspirations will become stifled. This leads to a feeling of being trapped which is often accompanied by a feeling of powerlessness; the result of this is usually a build-up of emotional pressure that eventually manifests as bursts of expressed anger. This is the Hun's way of letting off the pressure. If this anger is not released then the excess Liver Qi building up will instead begin to harm the rest of the body's internal organs and systems.

The Yin function of the Liver is to store the Blood. According to Daoist thought the Blood (or more importantly Ying Qi) is stored within the Liver until it is needed. During exercise more blood is passed to the muscles and tendons for nourishment and during periods of rest, including sleep, a great deal of Blood returns to the Liver for storage until needed. If the Liver's Yin function is not carried out successfully then problems will arise.

The Liver also governs the health of the tendons and sinews of the body.

Physical Manifestations

The Wood energy manifests as the organ of the liver when it reaches the physical realm. This energy also manifests within the nails of the fingers and toes.

Figure 7.8 summarises the various functions of the Liver.

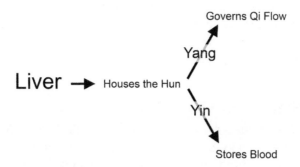

Figure 7.8: The Functions of the Liver

The Pericardium (Xin Bao)

The spiritual light of Fire divides into two Yin organs. The first is the Heart and the second is the Pericardium although a more accurate name for this organ is the Heart Protector.

The light of Fire has a strong link to the Heavens through its links to Shen and the space at the centre of the Heart. It is an energy which is easily affected by the movements of the emotions and interactions with others. Unhealthy emotional experiences would quickly bring damage to the Fire energy of the body and then in turn the Heart if it were not for the protection which the Pericardium offers. The spiritual role of the Heart Protector is to protect the Heart from damage; like a shield it takes negative information which is often passed on from others and protects the delicate Heart system. If the energy of the Pericardium becomes deficient then the Heart and Shen are more prone to emotional damage.

The spiritual energy of the Pericardium helps to govern the strength of a field of emotional information which expands out from the physical body at a distance of roughly 12 inches. This is the first line of defence against emotional 'attacks' from others. The health of our Fire energy, our Shen and our Qi along with the Pericardium govern the effectiveness of this protective layer.

The Yang (Fu) Organs

The Yang organs are not given the same level of importance within Daoist teachings as the Yin organs. This is because they are primarily seen as being in a supporting role to the Yin organs which have a more direct link to the five spiritual aspects of consciousness. For this reason the Yang organs are discussed here in less detail. Note though, that they are still formed in the same manner as the Yin organs: the spiritual energy of the five lights descends into the energetic realm and then manifests as an organ within the physical realm.

The Small Intestine (Xiao Chang)

The Small Intestine is the sorter of the pure from the impure. On a physical level this is seen in its role of taking food from the Stomach which it then divides into clean and turbid. The clean and useful elements of the food are distributed around the body while the turbid elements are sent to the Bladder and Large Intestine ready for expulsion from the body.

On a spiritual level the Small Intestine governs our ability to distinguish between thoughts and actions which are 'pure and impure'. This is the aspect of consciousness which enables us to decide between what are correct and healthy actions as opposed to those that are bad or unethical. An imbalance here can lead to a person having negative behaviour patterns and very little conscience. An extreme manifestation of this may be physically, verbally or sexually abusive tendencies.

The Stomach (Wei)

The Stomach's primary role is the 'rotting and ripening' of food matter. It works very closely with its paired organ, the Spleen. The Stomach takes the food and prepares it for the Spleen which then absorbs useful energy. Once this process is complete, the food is passed down into the Small Intestine ready for the sorting of the pure from the impure.

On a spiritual level the Stomach also helps us to digest ideas. Strong Stomach energy means that we are able to mentally absorb ideas and experiences and process them into something useful. Those with a weakness in the energy of the Stomach will find it very difficult to understand new concepts and learn from their experiences.

The Large Intestine (Da Chang)

The Large Intestine's role on a physical level is the same as understood within Western biological sciences. It takes matter which has no nutritional use for the body and expels it as faeces. Spiritually the Large Intestine also governs our ability to mentally let go.

The health of the Large Intestine dictates how well we are able to move past difficult experiences we have had and get on with our lives without these experiences haunting us. Just as the physical organ of the Large Intestine can become clogged with physical matter our minds can become clogged with past events. If the Large Intestine is not strong enough to let go of a sad past event or hurt that somebody has caused us then it is common for the paired Yin organ, the Lungs, to express this past event as sadness.

The Bladder (Pang Guang)

The Bladder governs the removal of fluid waste from the body through micturition. It is supported in this role by the Yang energy of the Kidneys which warm the Bladder and help it to hold the urine. If the Yang aspect of the Kidneys is weak then it is common for the Bladder to become weak. This can eventually lead to incontinence of urine.

The spiritual function of the Bladder is linked to the location of the Bladder meridian. This meridian is very long and runs across a person's back and over their head. It is akin to an energetic shield which protects the back of the body and the neck from invasion of pathogenic factors. When somebody is in extreme emotional distress it is common for them to curl up in a foetal position. This expands the Bladder meridian around the body in a protective manner. For this reason the spiritual aspect of the Bladder is linked to our own value or self-worth. A weakness in this organ will result in a person becoming insecure or lacking in confidence. The element of the Bladder is Water which is associated with the emotion of fear. Bladder imbalances manifest a sense of inner fear or fear of your own weaknesses.

The Gall Bladder (Dan)

The Gall Bladder receives bile from the Liver which it stores until needed for assistance in the process of digestion. In this way the function of the Gall Bladder according to Daoism matches the understanding of the gall bladder from a Western medical perspective.

The Gall Bladder is known as the 'decision maker'. This has two main meanings with regards to its energetic and spiritual functions. On an energetic level the Gall Bladder governs the decision making of the other Zang and Fu organs. As its paired organ, the Liver, governs the free-flow of Qi throughout the body, the Gall Bladder governs the way in which this energetic information is processed by the organs. If the Gall Bladder is weak then problems can also arise within any of the other organs. It is common within classical acupuncture treatments that the Gall Bladder is utilised alongside the rest of the treatment when the aim is to strengthen the function of any of the other organs.

On a spiritual level the Gall Bladder governs the strength of our decision making. A weakness in the Gall Bladder can manifest as a complete lack of ability when it comes to making even the most trivial decisions.

The Triple Heater (San Jiao)

The Triple Heater is an unusual concept for people new to Daoism to understand. It is an interesting aspect of the human body as unlike the rest of the Zang Fu it does not manifest physically. Although born from the spiritual light of Fire energy along with the Heart, Small Intestine and its paired organ, the Pericardium, the Triple Heater never develops beyond the energetic realm; it has no physical manifestation. Instead the Triple Heater is comprised of three energetic chambers which serve to regulate the internal pressures of the body as well as govern the flow of Jing, Qi, Shen, Blood and body fluids. Within contemporary Chinese medicine theory the Triple Heater is seen as three chambers that exist within the torso; these chambers dictate the level of harmony between the rest of the Yin and the Yang organs. Within Daoism this is a little different. The lower chamber of the Triple Heater sits below the diaphragm and is governed by the lower Dan Tien. The middle chamber sits above the diaphragm and is governed by the middle Dan Tien. The upper chamber is within the head and is governed by the upper Dan Tien. Figure 6.5 shows the location of the three chambers of the Triple Heater.

An imbalance within any one of the three chambers of the Triple Heater will manifest as problems with the Dan Tien or the organs within the area as well as possible issues with regards to fluid and energy flow.

Spiritually the Triple Heater governs our ability to hold non-romantic relationships with those around us. A weakness here will result in a person becoming withdrawn and unable to function socially.

The Extra Fu Organs

As well as the Yin and Yang organs there are also the six extra Fu organs which make up the final elements of Daoist physiology. They are different from the rest of the organs as they cannot be so easily categorised as either Yin (Zang) or Yang (Fu) organs. While they are like Yin organs in their close relationship to energies and essences they are also like Yang organs in that they are hollow.

The extra Fu organs are not usually given much importance at all within contemporary Chinese medicine practice but within classical Daoist theory they were an important part of the inner environment of the human body. Just like the rest of the body they are born forth first from consciousness, have an energetic presence and finally manifest as a physical organ.

The extra Fu organs are as follows:

- The Uterus
- The Brain
- The Marrow
- The Bones
- The Blood Vessels
- The Gall Bladder

The Uterus (Zi Bao)

As with the majority of ancient traditions, the feminine is seen as far closer to the divine than the masculine within Daoism. This is clear to see from the prevalence of goddess worship across the ancient world. Yin gives birth to Yang as absolute stillness gives birth to new life and movement. The Uterus is the most Yin of the organs of the body and recognised by Daoists as the bringer of new life.

Spiritual Attributes

The spiritual lights of Water and Wood work together within the female body to create the Uterus. The sinking down movement of Water provides a perfect base for the Yin energies of the Uterus to form while the shooting forth movement of Wood is the seed for the spark of new life. With regards to consciousness and the psyche, the Uterus provides a woman with a link to her own femininity. Not the disempowering image of femininity which holds sway within modern culture but rather the important role of the bringer of new life and mother to the next generation. This is the manifestation of the pivotal roles of Yin: birthing, protecting and nourishing.

As the Uterus has a close connection to the Kidneys it also brings a woman closer to the Zhi which resides there. The will of Heaven is stronger within women than men and the innate wisdom that resides deep within the centre of human consciousness is more easily tapped into by the female of the species. Imbalances with regards to how a woman perceives her role within society and as a woman can have a knock on effect to the Uterus and fertility in general.

Energetic Functions
The Yang function of the Uterus is to house the foetus during pregnancy. The energetic chamber of the Uterus is the receiver of the five spiritual lights of pure consciousness upon the conception of new life. It is also the location where the foetus develops as is understood within Western science.

The Yin function of the Uterus is to connect a woman to the energetic cycles of the moon. The moon is the Heavenly manifestation of pure Yin energy; a source of spiritual energy which governs not only the tides of the oceans but also the tides of energy moving through a person's body. While men are affected to some degree by the energy of the moon, women are closely linked to its cycles and movements.

The Moon Cycles
The moon orbits our planet in an anti-clockwise direction reflecting the light of the sun. The sun emits pure Yang energy via the rays of light which shine down onto the Earth. As the Yang energy of the sun is reflected off of the surface of the moon it becomes Yin and it is this frequency of energy which governs the flow of Qi and Blood strongly through the body. As the moon moves towards being full, Qi and Blood are stronger in the upper parts of our body. On a full moon the head is particularly full of Qi which is why those suffering with some kind of mental illness may find that it is worse on these days. As the moon moves away from being full, the Qi and Blood move downwards until on a new moon energy is very low in the body and people are more likely to be tired.

Figure 7.9 shows the phases of the moon in the Northern and Southern hemisphere and how these relate to the rising and falling of Qi and Blood within the body.

The energy of the moon governs several aspects of a person's health including fertility. Human beings, when in a balanced state, should be more fertile on a full moon. Traditionally, within Daoism, it was understood that the constitution of a child conceived during the build-up to, or ideally on, a full moon was much stronger. The Yin energy is more rooted and so the foundation of the Jing is more abundant. Conversely, children conceived upon a new moon tend to have weaker constitutions and be more prone to mental disturbances.

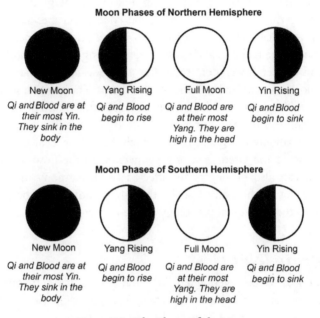

Figure 7.9: The Phases of the Moon

The reaction of the Uterus to the moon's cycles can be seen in the menstrual cycle. In a physically, energetically and emotionally balanced woman, menstruation should begin on a new moon. Qi and Blood are moving downwards and, as the Daoists say, the Heavenly Water can flow. This makes the menstruation process a healthy and cleansing experience. Ovulation should be in line with the full moon. Women are always closely governed by the waxing and waning of the moon, even when they have passed the age of having a menstrual cycle. According to Daoist teachings, negative side effects associated with the menopause in women are a sign of being energetically out of sync with the cycles of the moon for a protracted period of time. A classically trained acupuncturist may well want to treat various organ imbalances in this case but they may also want to carry out a treatment which brings you back in line with the influence of the moon's cycles.

If the Uterus is out of balance then premenstrual symptoms such as emotional disturbances will manifest. Emotional swings and physical pain, cramps and so forth are not supposed to be a part of the menstrual cycle; they are a sign that disharmony is present.

The Uterus and the Congenital Meridians

The congenital meridians have a strong link to the energy of the Uterus, in particular the governing meridian, the conception meridian and the thrusting meridian. These meridians also have a strong connection with the energy of the Kidneys and assist in transporting Jing, Qi and Blood to the Uterus to keep it well nourished. Any weakness in these meridians can have a knock on effect to the health of the Uterus. The governing meridian controls the Yang aspect of the Uterus's energetic function. The conception meridian controls the Yin aspect of the Uterus and the thrusting meridian governs the amount of Qi and Blood which the Uterus receives.

Because of the Uterus's strong connection to the flow of Blood in women it can also be negatively affected by disharmony in the Zang and Fu organs of the body. Usually though, pathology of the Uterus is included in the individual pathology of the relevant organs.

The Brain (Nao)

The Brain is often overlooked in Chinese medicine theory as an unimportant part of the human anatomy. The pervading view is that the ancient Chinese did not understand the brain very well so they omitted it from their theory. This is not true. The focus of Daoist thought, and so arts that came from this tradition such as Chinese medicine, is on the energetic realm. Although the physical body must be cared for and nurtured, the energy body is the target of most Daoist medicinal practices. Many of the functions which Western science would attribute to the brain are actually assigned to the Heart in Daoist philosophy because of its close links to the Shen, the monarch of human consciousness. Instead the Brain is seen as something like an organic filter.

When reality as we understand it is born from the great potential of Dao it moves down through the spiritual, energetic and, then finally, the physical realm. It is here that we all live and here that our body interacts with the world of matter. The physical realm is only one level of existence and a very low frequency realm at that. It is only a very small part of the great spectrum of existence and yet it is here, within this very small part of the spectrum that most people choose to define their world. Figure 7.10 illustrates this concept.

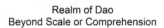

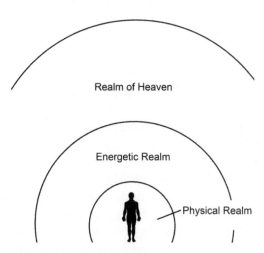

Figure 7.10: The Spectrum of Existence

It is the brain that connects us to this very small part of the spectrum of existence. If the brain did not carry out this role we would be bombarded with all of the information of reality at once. The physical world would be no more real to us than the energetic and the spiritual, and this amount of information would make it impossible for us to function; we would be driven insane. Luckily the Yang energetic function of the Brain is to filter out what is unnecessary so that this is not the case. Through Daoist alchemical practices we raise up the Shen to the upper Dan Tien which resides within the Brain. This enables the frequency of the Brain to adjust allowing different parts of the spectrum of existence to open up. The filter is changed to suit our needs and new levels of comprehension can be gained. The opening of the third eye which many spiritual traditions talk about achieves a similar goal. In Daoism this area is known as Yintang and it is shown in Figure 7.11.

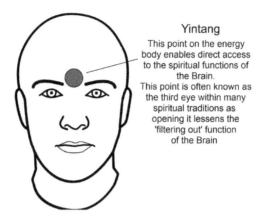

Figure 7.11: Yintang and the Brain

The Yin function of the brain is to process information which we receive from the outside world via our senses. It is for this reason that a weakness in the Yin aspect of the Brain can lead to deficiencies in sight, hearing, smell and so on. Within Chinese medicine theory sensory weaknesses are usually attributed to individual organs such as hearing to the Kidneys. This is, in part, due to the link between these organs and the Brain.

Some find it strange that the Brain has no meridian of its own. I would argue that it does, the governing meridian is the meridian of the Brain in the same way that the conception meridian is the primary meridian of the Uterus.

The Marrow (Sui)

The Marrow within Daoism is quite different from the bone marrow of Western science. This is, once again, an energetic substance which when manifested within the physical realm divides into the three substances of bone marrow, brain matter and the marrow of the spine. Figure 7.12 summarises the physical manifestations of the Marrow.

Marrow does not come from the spiritual realm. Instead it is born from the Jing; the essence of the Kidneys. From the Jing, the Marrow is created, it moves up through the spine into the brain and then manifests physically as the substances listed above; for this reason it has no major connections to the state of the psyche.

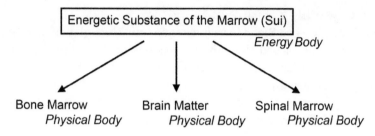

Figure 7.12: The Physical Manifestations of the Marrow

Weaknesses in the Marrow manifest as weaknesses of spinal posture and poor Brain function. A weakness here is usually due to a person being born with a predisposition to weakness in their Jing. This may be the result of poor health in the parents or genetic abnormalities.

The Bones (Gu)

The Bones are understood to be one of the extra Fu organs as they store the Marrow in the same way that the Yin organs store various vital substances.

The Bones are the support of the body. Like the Marrow, they are not born from the spiritual realm and instead grow from the same energy as the Kidneys. This link between Kidneys and Bones continues throughout our lifetime and weakness of the Kidneys will likely manifest as a Bone disorder. Aside from this, the Daoist understanding of the Bones is not so different from the Western medical understanding.

The Blood Vessels (Xue Mai)

The Blood Vessels are considered one of the extra Fu organs because they house the Blood. They are primarily governed by the Heart which controls their health and the Spleen which ensures that Blood remains flowing through the vessels. If the Spleen is weakened then it is possible for the Blood to leak from the vessels which results in internal haemorrhage and bruising.

As we have seen from our discussion of the Heart and its relationship to the Blood, Blood is the physical anchor for the Ying Qi and the Shen. Though the Shen is primarily housed within the space of the Heart, some of it also flows through the body via the blood. The Ying Qi nourishes the body with energy while the Shen provides a strong link between mind and body.

The Crystalline Nature of Blood

The Daoists viewed Blood in an interesting way. Through profound levels of inner vision gained through long periods of deep meditation they saw that Blood has a crystalline nature. The result of this is that as the energy of consciousness hits the blood via the Shen it splits up into its five component parts once more. The five lights manifest once again within the level of the Blood as shown in Figure 7.13.

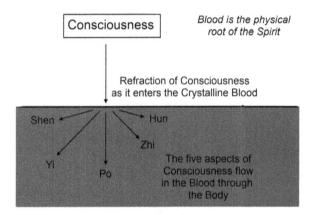

Figure 7.13: The Shen and the Blood

The five lights moving within the Blood mean that the Shen, Hun, Po, Yi and Zhi all have a strong presence within the Blood Vessels. The different aspects of human consciousness move in this manner through the physical body meaning that the level of balance and harmony within our psyche has a direct influence upon the entire body. Even a single thought has the power to change the health of our organs; this is one of the foundational principles upon which Chinese medicine was originally based. This fact carries great importance when we understand that the five spiritual aspects of consciousness that travel through the Blood are no more than manifestations of the five elemental energies. These five energies also manifest on an emotional level as the five emotions. Each of these five emotions has an impact upon the aspect of consciousness linked to it and the organs associated with that element. These are summarised in Table 7.2.

This means that any excessive emotions that a person experiences throughout their lives has a direct route via the Heart and the Shen into the Blood which then divides and reaches the relevant organs. For this reason it is important that we seek to balance our emotional state which will in turn protect our health. From a Daoist perspective it also means that treating the Blood can help to balance a person's emotional state.

Table 7.2: Emotions, Spirits and Organs

	Fire	Earth	Metal	Water	Wood
Spirit	Shen	Yi	Po	Zhi	Hun
Emotion	Excitation	Worry	Sadness	Fear	Anger
Yin Organ	Heart and Small Intestine	Spleen	Lungs	Kidneys	Liver
Yang Organ	Pericardium and Triple Heater	Stomach	Large Intestine	Bladder	Gall Bladder

Qi and Blood

Qi is Yang, it is energy, it is information. Blood is Yin, it is substance, it is nourishment. These two work closely together as they move through the body. The result of this is that both Qi and Blood need to be healthy in order to maintain harmony within the body. The Qi propels the Blood through the body by providing it with a motive force. The Blood supports the Qi and in particular Ying Qi which it, in turn, carries. If Qi becomes deficient then it can no longer propel the Blood which will then become stagnant which results in pain and imbalance. If the Blood is deficient then it can no longer carry the Ying Qi and so the energy body will not receive the nourishment that it needs to function. This is an important reflection of the harmonious relationship which needs to exist between Yin and Yang on multiple levels within the body.

The Gall Bladder (Dan)

The Gall Bladder is somewhat of an anomaly as it appears within the Yang (Fu) organs and the extra Fu organs. It appears within the extra Fu organs because of its function of storing bile which the Liver produces. Also, it does not deal with food matter or waste like the rest of the Yang (Fu) organs which makes it fairly unique.

As the Gall Bladder has been discussed above it will not be explored in further detail here.

Interaction of the Zang Fu Organs: One System

Western medical science understands living creatures as being comprised of numerous systems such as the respiratory system, the nervous system and so on. The Daoist view of the body differs in that it considers there only to be one system; this is the system of the body.

It is beyond the scope of this book to go into great detail covering the inter-relations of the various organs of the body; it would be best to refer to a detailed Chinese medicine textbook to read about these interactions in detail. Instead I have summarised the relationship between the various organs in the following three diagrams. Figure 7.14 shows the relationships of the Yin (Zang) organs; Figure 7.15 shows the relationships of the Yang (Fu) organs and Figure 7.16 puts these together with the extra Fu organs into one complete system.

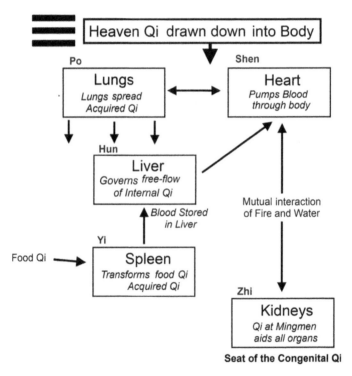

Figure 7.14: Yin Organ Relationships

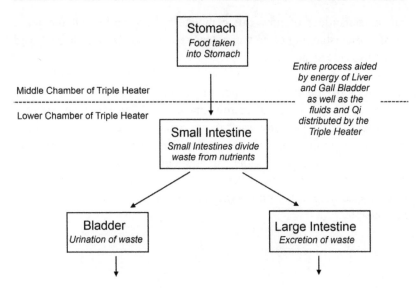

Figure 7.15: Yang Organ Relationships

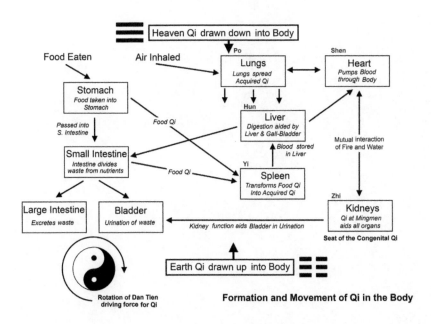

Figure 7.16: The Whole Body System

An understanding of how this complete system works will provide a greater understanding of how imbalance takes place within the body and how this leads to sickness.

It is recommended that you spend a fair amount of time familiarising yourself with the functions and interactions of the Zang Fu organs which have been discussed in this chapter, as they will enable you to understand how your body reacts to the changes which take place within your inner environment throughout your life. The more familiar you are able to become with the various Yin and Yang functions of the different organs discussed here, the easier it will be to understand the nature of disease according to the philosophy of Daoism which is looked at in the next chapter.

CHAPTER 8

DISRUPTION OF HEAVEN AND EARTH

Heaven exerts a strong energetic force downwards into the body; this is the extreme manifestation of the power of Yang. From below we receive the power of Yin via the energetic influence of the Earth. We live between these two forces, receivers for the information which meets within us. As the forces of Yin and Yang intermingle in an ever shifting swirl of energy within our body we experience the various processes of life, growth and evolution. The Daoist way is to remain open to these forces and to simply go with the flow. Cultivate emptiness within so that Heaven and Earth may move through us and we may benefit from their influence. As with many things that are good for us, however, remaining empty is a difficult state to maintain and consequently we shift, to varying degrees, out of balance with the two poles. The result is disharmony which leads to sickness.

In order to evolve spiritually through practice of the internal arts we must first build the strongest foundation we can with regards to our health. In order to build this foundation and improve our health we must first understand the signs of poor health and the nature of sickness according to the Daoist tradition. What follows now is a summary of the most common internal imbalances that may take place within the Yin and Yang organs of the body. A list of the common symptoms is given as well as a commentary explaining the reason for these symptoms appearing.

Zang Fu Disturbances

Whether or not the sickness is caused internally or externally, at some point in the development of disease there will likely be an effect on the Zang and Fu organs of the body. Here, only the most common of the disturbances which may affect the organs of the body are listed. Within the Chinese medical tradition diagnosis of the organs usually falls under one of the headings listed within this chapter. This means that your diagnosis may be something like: Spleen Qi Deficiency or Liver Yang rising. Study this chapter to understand the nature of energetic imbalance once it reaches the level of the organs.

Heart (Xin) Disturbances

The most common imbalances of the Heart are: Heart Yin deficiency, Heart Yang deficiency, Heart Qi deficiency, Heart Blood deficiency, Heart Fire and Heart Blood Stagnation. These are discussed below.

Heart Yin Deficiency

Classical signs of Heart Yin deficiency are:

- mental agitation
- sweating on the palms of the hand and the soles of the feet
- excessive sweating at night.

The Yin energetic function of the Heart governs the energetic strength of the Blood via the Ying Qi. Since Blood is the physical anchor for the spiritual energy of the Shen, a weakness in the quality of the Blood because of weak Heart Yin energy will mean that the Shen is 'un-rooted'. The result is that the consciousness becomes disturbed resulting in mental agitation.

Yin is cooling while Yang is warming. If the Heart's Yin aspect is weak the Heart will warm up due to its Yang aspect being unchecked. The Heart does not like being excessively hot and so it will try to vent excess heat from the body via the palms and soles. The reason for this is because of the meridian points: Kidney 1 (Yongquan) and Pericardium 8 (Laogong) which are major exit points for heat from the body. Figure 8.1 shows the location of these points. As heat escapes the body it will cause this area to start sweating.

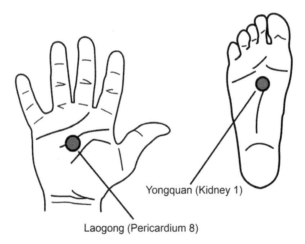

Yongquan (Kidney 1)

Laogong (Pericardium 8)

Figure 8.1: Exit Points for Internal Heat

The night time is Yin in comparison to the day which is Yang. The body reflects this and at night goes into a more Yin state than during the day. The energy stills, mental activity lessens and the body gets ready for rest. If the Heart's Yin function is weak then there will be an excess of heat in the Heart. This excess heat will prevent the body from going into a fully Yin state so it will try to expel the heat from the body. The result is excessive sweating at night.

Heart Yang Deficiency

Classical signs of Heart Yang deficiency are:

- cold hands and feet

- excessive sweating which is not time specific

- feeling emotionally drained.

The Yang energetic function of the Heart is to propel the Blood through the vessels of the body. This Blood provides warmth throughout the body; if the Blood is not propelled efficiently enough then the extremities will constantly feel cold no matter how warm the weather. According to Chinese medical thought the Blood and the body's sweat have a close relationship. If there is too much Blood it will transform into sweat to prevent there being an excessive build-up. The Blood is not being propelled in this condition so it transforms into excessive sweating which is often cold in nature.

Heart Qi Deficiency

Classical signs of Heart Qi deficiency are:

- palpitations or irregular heart-beat

- shortness of breath

- excessive sweating

- tiredness

- low mood.

If an organ is Qi deficient it means that the energy of the organ is weak. This will affect all energetic functions of the body with no emphasis on either Yin or Yang.

The Heart's energy is weak so the physical organ is also affected which will result in palpitations and an irregular heart-beat. Because of the close relationship that exists between the Heart and the Lungs there will also be a shortness of breath and a tight chest. It is said within classical Daoism that if the Shen is disturbed by a weakness of the Heart, the Po will begin to struggle resulting in the Lungs becoming weak.

The lack of ability to propel the Blood through the body will mean that there is too much Blood backed up around the body so it will begin to transform into sweat; this ensures that stagnation does not occur. This sweat can come at any time and is not dependent on times of the day or amount of physical exertion.

If the Heart's energy is weak, Ying Qi and Blood will not reach the rest of the body which will result in tiredness. This will also cause the Fire energy of the Heart to burn dimly. There will be a lack of excitation which results in a low mood and despondence.

Heart Blood Deficiency

Classical signs of Heart Blood deficiency are:

- insomnia and dream-disturbed sleep

- pale face and lips

- dizziness.

If the Blood is deficient then the Shen is not held in place. The consciousness is not rooted in the Blood and reaching the rest of the body; instead it moves freely outside of the vessels. The result is that during the night the consciousness becomes disturbed. The Shen has too strong a connection with information from Heaven which results in excessive dreaming and disturbed sleep.

If there is a deficiency of Blood the face and lips become pale as the head is not nourished properly; this will also result in dizziness.

Heart Fire

Classical signs of Heart Fire are:

- mental agitation and insomnia

- red face

- mouth ulcers, particularly on the tongue.

The heart does not like excessive heat. If there is too much heat here then it is known as Heart Fire. This imbalance is almost always rooted in the consciousness. Excessive emotional disturbances have filled the emptiness within the centre of the Heart. The Shen is disturbed and mental agitation is the result. Too much expansion of the Fire Qi of the Heart causes heat to rise to the head resulting in a flushed face. A person with this condition will become overly excitable as the Fire Qi takes over the control of their emotional nature.

The energy of Fire Qi manifests within the physical realm not only as the organ of the heart but also the tongue. Excess heat will move up to the tongue resulting in mouth ulcers.

Heart Blood Stagnation

Classical signs of Heart Blood stagnation are:

- stabbing pain in the chest which moves down the left arm
- stiff neck
- tight chest.

If Blood stagnates around the Heart then excessive energetic blockages are the result. This is extremely dangerous and immediate help should be sought out. The excessive build-up of Blood means that the Heart's energy cannot flow as it needs to. There will be a sharp stabbing pain in the area of the physical heart which often travels down the left arm along the line of the Heart meridian. The chest is also tight along with the neck due to the pathway of the internal branches of the Heart meridian.

This is a dangerous level of internal imbalance as the physical manifestation of this condition is usually a heart attack.

Spleen (Pi) Disturbances

The most common imbalances of the Spleen are: Spleen Yang deficiency, Spleen Qi deficiency and Cold in the Spleen. These are discussed below.

Spleen Yang Deficiency

Classical signs of Spleen Yang deficiency are:

- pale face
- cold arms and legs
- poor appetite
- abdominal swelling after eating.

Yang is warming so if this aspect of the Spleen's energy is weak it will mean that the body becomes cold. The muscles of the arms, legs, hands and feet will be particularly cold as the heat from the body cannot reach the extremities.

The lack of warmth in the body will cause a pale face as the Spleen is also traditionally understood to help keep the Blood within the vessels of the body. This blood will not reach the uppermost parts of the body. Remember that the Yang function of the Spleen is to uplift; if Yang is deficient then energy will sink away from the head.

If the Yang function of the Spleen is weakened then Qi drawn from the food will not be sent upwards for further processing by the other organs. The result is that the abdomen will swell due to a build-up of food energy; this swelling is worse after eating as it takes time for the Spleen to struggle to send the energy upwards.

Spleen Qi Deficiency
Classical signs of Spleen Qi deficiency are:

- yellow complexion
- abdominal swelling
- diarrhoea
- sinking energy in the abdomen
- an inability to focus.

The colour of Earth energy is yellow. Since the Earth energy of the body governs the Spleen, a strong imbalance in this organ will manifest as a slightly yellow tinge to a person's skin.

The Qi of the Spleen is weak in this condition. This weakness has no leaning towards either Yin or Yang. All functions of the Spleen will be negatively affected including the Yang function of raising the Qi and the function of transforming the food into usable energy by the body. The weak Yang function results in abdominal swelling and a feeling of the abdomen sinking downwards. In extreme cases this sinking of Qi results in the prolapse of organs.

The weak Spleen Qi function means that the food is not processed properly by the Spleen which results in diarrhoea and sometimes constipation. Much of the useful energy is not removed from the food prior to the waste entering the large intestines. The result of this is that after a protracted period of deficient Spleen Qi a person will become malnourished.

Cold in the Spleen
Classical signs of Cold in the Spleen are:

- swelling in the abdomen
- heavy feeling throughout the body and limbs
- diarrhoea.

The Spleen does not like to be cold. This condition is usually caused by an external condition of Cold moving deep into the body and affecting the Spleen on an energetic level. The Cold entering the Spleen causes its function of absorbing energy from the food to go into hypo-function (reduced function). The result is a thick build-up of Qi around the body which was known as Damp within Daoist medical sciences.

The excess Cold Damp in the body causes the abdomen to swell and the limbs to feel heavy as if they are sponges soaked in water. Moving is a lot of effort and the muscles are weak.

The lack of energy being drawn from the food prior to entering the Large Intestine results in diarrhoea which is also a sign of internal Cold in Chinese medicine.

Lung (Fei) Disturbances

The most common imbalances of the Lungs are: Lung Yin deficiency, Lung Qi deficiency, Wind invasion of the Lungs and Phlegm in the Lungs. These are discussed below.

Lung Yin Deficiency
Classical signs of Lung Yin deficiency are:

- dry cough, sometimes with blood
- high body temperature in the afternoon
- depression/low mood.

The Yin function of the lungs is to govern the dispersal of body fluids throughout the body. These fluids moisten everything as well as carrying out numerous other functions. If the Yin of the Lungs becomes deficient then they will dry up resulting in a dry cough. In extreme cases this may lead to a cough which produces blood.

The afternoon is the time of day when Yang energy starts to switch into Yin energy. As the body moves into a Yin state excess heat will show up clearly resulting in a high body temperature or fever in the afternoon. This is only present in protracted periods of Lung Yin deficiency.

Lung Qi Deficiency
Classical signs of Lung Qi deficiency are:

- weak cough
- difficulty breathing or weak breathing
- weak voice
- spontaneous sweating.

In this condition the energy of the Lungs is weak with no emphasis on either Yin or Yang. The weak function of the Lungs will result in a weak cough and difficulty breathing. The breathing will be shallow and sometimes a little laboured. This is very common and often the person with weak Lung Qi will be totally unaware of the poor quality of their breathing until it is pointed out to them.

There is an interesting concept concerning the voice in classical Daoist mythology. The Lungs are said to be like a cave in which the spirit of the Po lives. This mournful spirit expresses himself by shouting and allowing the sounds to echo from the inside of the caves where he lives. This echoing expression of the Po is your voice; if the Lungs' Qi is weak then the caves do not echo very well. This means that the sound of the Po shouting is lessened, the result is a weak voice. Figure 8.2 summarises this concept.

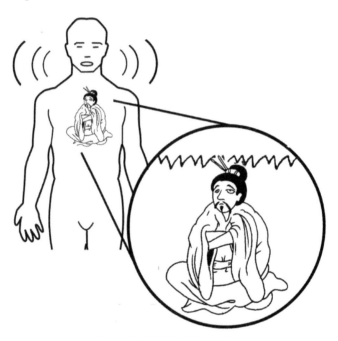

Figure 8.2: The Po in his Cave

Although this is just a story to illustrate the reason for weakness of voice being associated with deficient Lung Qi it is still a useful way to remember the link between the two.

Wind Invasion of the Lungs

Classical signs of Wind invading the Lungs are:

- cough with either yellow or white sputum

- thirst or absence of thirst

- headache

- nasal blockage

- tight or sore throat.

External Wind usually attacks the Lungs before any other organ due to the Lungs having a direct opening to the outside environment via the mouth and throat. They were classically considered the most sensitive organ of the Zang Fu for this reason.

Wind may produce either one of two effects when it affects the Lungs. It will either produce hot or cold symptoms. When the Lungs are attacked a cough will always be present. Cold Wind will mean that a person coughs up white sputum while a hot Wind will produce yellow sputum. Whether or not a person is thirsty will also indicate the temperature of the Wind invasion with heat causing a strong thirst and cold preventing a person from feeling thirsty. Hot Wind will also produce a sore throat while cold Wind will result in a tight throat.

A headache is common when Wind invades the Lungs as the Wind also often attacks the meridians which run across the face and head.

Phlegm in the Lungs

Classical signs of Phlegm in the Lungs are:

- tight, difficult breathing

- tightness in the chest

- phlegm production when coughing.

When the Lungs are weakened the energy will stagnate there. Stagnant Qi often produces Phlegm in the body and the Lungs are particularly prone to a build-up of Phlegm.

Excess Phlegm in the Lungs will mean that breathing becomes difficult and the throat/chest often feels tight. Phlegm, as understood within Western science, is also produced when the person coughs.

Kidney (Shen) Disturbances

The most common imbalances of the Kidneys are: Kidney Yin deficiency, Kidney Yang deficiency and Kidney Qi deficiency. These are discussed below. The Kidneys are a particularly important organ to understand from an internal arts perspective as imbalances within the Kidneys often have an immediate and strong knock on effect to the other organs of the body.

Kidney Yin Deficiency

Classical signs of Kidney Yin deficiency are:

- weak back and knees
- dizziness and ringing in the ears
- poor memory
- nocturnal emissions
- dry mouth.

The key sign of any Kidney weakness is a weak back and knees. An internal branch of the Kidney meridian runs through the lower back as shown in Figure 8.3.

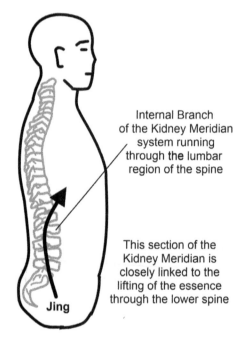

Figure 8.3: Internal Branch of the Kidney Meridian

If the Kidneys become deficient then the energy in this meridian is drained and so the spaces between the lumbar vertebrae of the spine will shrink. The result is weakness and lower back pain. The external Kidney meridian runs through the knees and these too will become weakened by a deficiency of Qi in this part of the body.

Since Yin is cooling, a deficiency of Yin will cause Yang to become excessive. Yang is heating and rising in nature so energy will move up towards the head. The ears are closely linked to the Kidneys so ringing in the ears is common along with spells of dizziness.

The Kidneys also have a close relationship to the Brain so deficiency here will bring about weakness of the Brain's functions including short term memory. In Daoism, short term memory is linked to the Brain while long term memory is linked to the Heart.

The Yin energetic function of the Kidneys is linked to our sexuality and reproduction in adult life. If this is weakened then, in extreme cases, there will be nocturnal leakage of sexual fluids which are often unaccompanied by dreams. In lesser cases of Kidney Yin deficiency there is a low sex drive instead.

Kidney Yang Deficiency

The classical signs of Kidney Yang deficiency are:

- weak back and knees
- pale skin
- cold extremities.

The Kidney's Yang function is linked closely to the Ming Fire which warms the body and causes the whole body system to function. If the Yang aspect of the Kidneys is weak then a person will feel cold and have a pale complexion. Note that they will also have the weak and sore back and knees which is characteristic of all Kidney deficiencies.

Kidney Qi Deficiency

Classical signs of Kidney Qi deficiency are:

- weak back and knees
- frequent urination
- premature ejaculation/difficulty reaching orgasm.

When the energy of the Kidneys is weak then its function of aiding the Bladder in storage of urine is compromised. This will mean that a person has to urinate frequently; often this continues throughout the night resulting either in night time urinary incontinence or waking to use the toilet. It is interesting to note that the Kidneys do not like the cold as this has a negative effect on the Ming Fire. If the lower back becomes cold then the Kidneys' Qi will weaken resulting in the above signs.

If the Kidneys' energy is also disturbed then they cannot hold the sexual fluids in place and men will suffer from premature ejaculation. In women this may manifest as difficulty reaching orgasm during sexual intercourse.

Liver (Gan) Disturbances

The most common imbalances of the Liver are: Liver Yin deficiency, Liver Qi stagnation, Liver Blood deficiency, Liver Blood stasis, Liver Yang rising and Liver Fire. These are discussed below.

Liver Yin Deficiency

Classical signs of Liver Yin deficiency are:

- dry eyes and blurred vision
- pale complexion but with flushed cheeks
- dizziness
- depression.

The Yin energetic function of the Liver is to store the Blood. If this is deficient then Blood will not reach the upper part of the body when needed, resulting in dry eyes and blurred vision. These are signs of a lack of Blood not moistening the body and the eyes are closely linked to the Liver. This is also the reason for dizziness; there is not enough Blood to reach the head.

The lack of Blood will cause the face to become pale but it is worth noting that the cheeks are still often flushed red. This is because of the cooling nature of Yin; if this is deficient then there will be too much heat produced within the Liver. Heat rises meaning that it will reach the head and produce the flushed cheeks.

Depression is due to a lack of Wood Qi. Wood is controlled by Metal within the five element theory. If the Wood is weak then the Metal becomes stronger; it continues to over-control or oppress the Wood Qi and so the emotion of Metal is dominant; this emotion is sadness which manifests as depression.

Liver Qi Stagnation

Classical signs of Liver Qi stagnation are:

- a feeling of tightness in the chest
- irritability
- melancholy
- pre-menstrual tension.

If the energy of the Liver becomes stagnant then Qi cannot flow efficiently throughout the body. This is the Yang energetic function of the Liver. The result of stagnant Qi caused by Liver Qi stagnation is a feeling of tightness in the chest which is accompanied by irritability, frustration and a sense of melancholy.

Women are prone to pre-menstrual tension symptoms that fluctuate between sadness and bursts of anger.

When your internal energy is stagnant this is not a nice feeling. It is restrictive and frustrating; many times when a person with stagnant Liver Qi cannot pinpoint any specific symptoms they will still express a feeling of being stuck. If the Liver Qi has been stagnant for some time then the Wood Qi causes a person to have anger management problems.

Liver Blood Deficiency

Classical signs of Liver Blood deficiency are:

- floaters in the eyes
- pale complexion
- dizziness
- depression
- scanty menstrual blood.

If the Liver Blood is deficient then the eyes begin to dry up which results in floaters appearing in the eyes. This is the key sign of Liver Blood deficiency. The lack of Blood reaching the face means that there will be a pale complexion; unlike Liver Yin deficiency there is not an excess of Yang energy so there is no heat rising to flush the cheeks.

The lack of Blood reaching the head leads to dizziness and the balance of Wood against Metal energy according to the theory of five elements leads to depression.

Women will also find that they have scanty menstrual blood and in extreme cases may not menstruate at all.

Liver Blood Stasis

Classical signs of Liver Blood stasis are:

- hypochondria and abdominal pain
- vomiting blood
- painful periods with clotting
- a feeling of inner frustration.

When Liver Blood stagnates in the body it can cause pain in the abdomen and hypochondriac region. This is sometimes accompanied by swelling and abdominal masses although this does not always have to be the case. Liver Blood stagnation is primarily a dysfunction of the Yang energetic function of the Liver as the Qi which moves with the Blood has been affected. This causes the Blood to stagnate. The reason it is not called Liver Yang deficiency is that it does not come with cold signs as the Yin does not move into excess. This is largely due to the warm nature of the stagnant Blood.

In extreme cases a person may vomit Blood.

Women often experience abdominal pain prior to their period starting and clotted blood during menstruation.

Liver Yang Rising

Classical signs of Liver Yang rising are:

- temporal headache
- eye pain
- dizziness
- dry mouth and throat
- anger outbursts.

When the Liver energy moves into excess it moves upwards through the body generating excess heat. This is usually the result of emotional strain affecting the Liver and for this reason Liver Yang rising is rarely the result of external pathogens.

As the Liver Yang Qi rises it moves into the head, building up pressure which results in migraine type headaches within the temporal regions of the head. The heat created here also causes eye pain, dizziness and a dry mouth and throat as the fluids are burnt up.

The negative emotion of Wood energy which governs the Liver is anger and so when the Liver is in excess there will be outbursts of anger.

The strength of this anger will depend upon the extent and duration of the condition.

Liver Fire

Classical signs of Liver Fire are:

- irritability
- strong outbursts of anger
- temporal headache
- dizziness
- red face and eyes
- nosebleeds.

Liver Yang rising will, over time, develop into Liver Fire which is a more extreme manifestation of the same excessive condition. The signs for Liver Fire are broadly the same as for Liver Yang rising with the exception that the outbursts of anger will be much stronger, often leading to violence. The excess heat will cause the face and eyes to become red and the heat in the Liver Blood may cause the Blood to 'over-boil' resulting in nosebleeds.

Pericardium (Xin Bao) Disturbances

The most common imbalances of the Pericardium are: Pericardium Qi stagnation and Pericardium Heat. These are discussed below. Note that the Pericardium is rarely considered within contemporary Chinese medicine practice despite that fact that both of the Pericardium conditions listed here are fairly commonplace.

Pericardium Qi Stagnation

Classical signs of Pericardium Qi stagnation are:

- a feeling of oppression in the chest
- slight shortness of breath
- sighing and a feeling of sadness.

The Pericardium protects the Heart from emotional damage. Its meridian has an external branch to the outside of the chest and an internal branch that runs to the heart as shown in Figure 8.4.

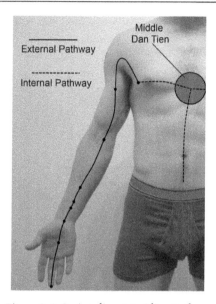

Figure 8.4: Pericardium Meridian Pathway

The Pericardium Qi usually stagnates during the early stages of emotional distress. The chest becomes tight and the breathing can become a little laboured. A person will have a feeling of sadness and begin to sigh or gasp for breath. This condition is clear to see when a person receives unexpected, sad news. It is also common for them to automatically reach up and touch the area of their Heart.

Pericardium Heat
Classical signs of Pericardium Heat are:

- a feeling of oppression in the chest
- hot feeling in body but cold hands and feet
- mental confusion with incoherent speech
- sighing.

Pericardium Qi stagnation may progress onto Pericardium Heat. This is the progression of sudden emotional trauma which the Pericardium is still preventing from reaching the Heart. The tight chest of Pericardium Qi stagnation is still present along with occasional sighing or gasping for breath; this sounds similar to somebody who has been swimming underwater who reaches the surface and gasps for air.

The heat in the Pericardium causes the body to become hot but it is almost as if the heat has been drawn in from the extremities which are still cold. The heat around the Pericardium affects the Shen which results in incoherent thoughts and speech.

This condition only comes from severe emotional shock. If the Pericardium is functioning well then it is generally short lived.

Yang (Fu) Organs

Pathology of the Yang organs is not discussed in as much detail as for the Yin organs in Chinese medical thought. Many symptoms associated with pathology of the Yang organs are instead grouped with their paired Yin organs as treatment here is often more efficient. For this reason the Yang organs are only discussed briefly.

Small Intestine (Xiao Chang) Disturbances

The most common imbalances of the Small Intestines are: Heat in the Small Intestines and Small Intestine Qi deficiency. These are discussed below.

Heat in the Small Intestines

Classical signs of Heat in the Small Intestines are:

- abdominal pain which feels hot
- tongue ulcers
- dark urination
- compromised ability to discriminate.

The key sensation of an uncomfortable heat in the lower abdomen which is accompanied with dark urination is the clearest sign of this condition. Tongue ulcers generally appear in chronic cases of this imbalance as does difficulty discriminating between good and bad ideas which is due to the spiritual function of the Small Intestines.

Small Intestine Qi Deficiency

Classical signs of Small Intestine Qi deficiency are:

- dull abdominal pain which feels bruised
- gurgling sounds in lower abdomen
- diarrhoea which often comes quickly after eating
- cold limbs.

If the Small Intestine Qi is deficient then there will be signs of Cold in the lower abdomen. Conversely it is also possible for Cold to invade the lower abdomen which will result in the Qi of the Small Intestines becoming weak. The food will not be held and processed effectively within the small intestines and so diarrhoea is the result. The dull abdominal pain is often helped with pressure; this is usually a clear sign of Qi deficiency.

Stomach (Wei) Disturbances

The most common imbalances of the Stomach are as follows: Damp Heat in the Stomach and Stomach Fire. These are discussed below.

Damp Heat in the Stomach

Classical signs of Damp Heat in the Stomach are:

- swelling in the abdomen and epigastrium
- nausea
- body feeling heavy and tired
- possible vomiting.

If Damp Heat has made its way into the Stomach, its function of 'rotting and ripening' will be disturbed. The natural flow of the Stomach's energy will also be affected meaning that Qi will rise resulting in possible vomiting. Damp is always accompanied by a feeling of being weighed down.

Stomach Fire

Classical signs of Stomach Fire are:

- burning pain in epigastrium
- sour tasting regurgitation
- large appetite
- ulcers
- bleeding gums.

The Stomach controls the level of our appetite; if it becomes too hot through an excessive type imbalance then our appetite will increase. This is accompanied by an uncomfortable feeling of warmth in the area of the stomach and signs of heat rising such as bleeding gums and mouth ulcers. As the Stomach Qi rises it will also cause sour tasting regurgitation which often leaves a feeling of warmth in the throat.

Large Intestine (Da Chang) Disturbances

The most common imbalances of the Large Intestine are as follows: Damp Heat in the Large Intestines and Dry Large Intestines. These are discussed below.

Damp Heat in the Large Intestines

Classical signs of Damp Heat in the Large Intestines are:

- abdominal pain
- bloody stools
- yellow diarrhoea
- burning anus.

If Damp Heat makes its way into the Large Intestines this will cause a burning pain in the lower abdomen along with yellow diarrhoea and a burning anus.

Dry Large Intestines

Classical signs of Dry Large Intestines are:

- constipation and dry stools
- foul breath.

If there is not enough fluid within the Large Intestines then their function becomes deficient. Constipation is the key sign along with dry stools. This is usually the result of another organ being affected so there will likely be other symptoms present. Due to the lack of fluids and the pairing of the Large Intestines with the Lungs there is often foul smelling breath as well.

Bladder (Pang Guang) Disturbances

The most common imbalances of the Bladder are as follows: Damp Heat in the Bladder and Deficient Bladder Qi. These are discussed below.

Damp Heat in the Bladder

Classical signs of Damp Heat in the Bladder are:

- frequent urination with a sense of urgency
- burning pain in urethra
- yellow urine.

As Damp Heat attacks the Bladder there will be frequent, yellow urine which is usually accompanied with pain.

Deficient Bladder Qi

Classical signs of deficient Bladder Qi are:

- frequent pale urination or difficulty urinating
- a feeling of discomfort in the urethra
- a sense of insecurity or low self-esteem.

This is often linked to a disorder of the Kidneys as they directly govern the function of the Bladder. Insecurity here is linked to the spiritual function of the Bladder.

Gall Bladder (Dan) Disturbances

The most common imbalances of the Gall Bladder are as follows: Damp in the Gall Bladder and Gall Bladder Qi deficiency. These are discussed below.

Damp in the Gall Bladder

Classical signs of Damp in the Gall Bladder are:

- dull headache with a feeling of pressure
- a sense of being swollen in the hypochondria
- feeling of heaviness in the body.

Due to the pathway of the Gall Bladder meridian, which is shown in Figure 8.5, Damp in the Gall Bladder will usually present with a dull headache. This feels as though the head is being squeezed. Damp always comes with a feeling of heaviness in the body which often results in feeling tired as well.

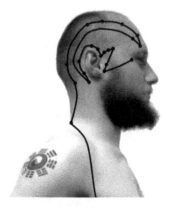

Figure 8.5: Gall Bladder Meridian

Gall Bladder Qi Deficiency

Classical signs of Gall Bladder Qi deficiency are:

- shyness
- lack of ability to make decisions.

Due to the spiritual function of the Gall Bladder a weakness of Gall Bladder Qi will result in an inability to make decisions. The Gall Bladder is also linked to confidence so deficient energy here will result in a person being timid.

Triple Heater (San Jiao) Disturbances

The most common disturbances of the Triple Heater are as follows: Upper Jiao Weakness, Middle Jiao Weakness, Lower Jiao Weakness and Triple Heater Qi Deficiency. These are discussed below. Please note that the conditions of the Triple Heater according to Daoism are very different from the conditions as understood within contemporary Chinese medicine. This is because of the traditional link of the San Jiao to the three Dan Tien, an understanding which has not been carried across into modern times.

Upper Jiao Weakness

Classical signs of Upper Jiao Weakness are:

- disturbed thinking processes
- unwanted thoughts.

The Triple Heater is divided into three sections known as the three Jiao. These are shown in Figure 6.5.

Each of these Jiao is linked to one of the three Dan Tien as shown. If the energy in one of the three Jiao becomes disturbed then the function of the Dan Tien linked to this Jiao will also be disturbed. If the upper Jiao is affected then it is common for a person's thoughts to become disturbed, often with unwanted imagery. These thoughts and images run at a fast pace through the mind and can be very tiring as well as distracting.

Middle Jiao Weakness

Classical signs of Middle Jiao Weakness are:

- strong emotional swings
- fixation on an emotional state.

If the middle Jiao is affected then the emotional centre becomes disturbed. A person with this condition will begin to swing from one heightened emotional state to another. One second they may be violently angry before becoming tearful and then laughing excitedly. There is often no catalyst for their emotional switches and they will present as very irrational.

Due to the link between the middle Dan Tien and the Heart, which houses the Shen, it is also likely that a person becomes fixed upon their emotional state. They will strongly identify with how they are feeling to an unhealthy degree. The middle Jiao is particularly affected by feelings of worthlessness and depression. It is common for people to become so connected to this state that their low emotional state becomes an ingrained part of their identity.

Lower Jiao Weakness

Classical signs of Lower Jiao weakness are:

- constant low energy despite looking after your health
- difficulty waking in the mornings.

The functions of the lower Jiao are linked to the lower Dan Tien and the Kidneys. Usually a person will look to the Kidneys first to treat the symptoms of unexplained tiredness and difficulty getting started in the mornings. If these symptoms persist, even with treatment and lifestyle changes then it may be a weakness in the energy of the lower Jiao.

Triple Heater Qi Deficiency

Classical signs of Triple Heater Qi deficiency are:

- multiple organ hypo (reduced) function
- low energy levels
- difficulty socialising.

The energy of the three Jiao together govern the actions of the body's organs. If the energy of the Triple Heater is deficient then these functions may go into hypo-function; there will be deficiency signs of several organs at the same time. The body will also be tired. Due to the spiritual function of the Triple Heater difficulty socialising or even leaving the house is often linked to a weakness of the Triple Heater.

Uterus (Zi Bao) Disturbances

The most common imbalances of the Uterus are as follows: Uterus Yang Deficiency, Uterus Yin Deficiency and Cold in the Uterus. These are discussed below.

Uterus Yang Deficiency

The classical sign of Uterus Yang deficiency is:

- a tendency towards miscarriages.

In contemporary Chinese medicine a tendency towards miscarriages is often linked to the health of other Zang Fu organs such as the Kidneys, Spleen and Liver. This is because treatment is most effective if focused upon the meridians of these organs along with the conception meridian. In traditional Daoist medicine the Uterus's Yang function helps to house the foetus during pregnancy so a weakness of its Yang function would lead to miscarriage. Any attempt to correct this imbalance would focus primarily on the conception meridian with support from the organ meridians. This is due to the fact that, in essence, the conception meridian is the Uterus meridian (in women).

Uterus Yin Deficiency

The classical signs of Yin deficiency is:

- lack of synchronicity with the moon's cycles.

As discussed previously, the Yin energetic function of the Uterus brings a woman into synchronicity with the movements of the moon. If a woman's menstrual cycle is not in time with the movements of the moon then this can be a sign of Uterus Yin deficiency.

Cold in the Uterus

Classical signs of Cold in the Uterus are:

- difficulty becoming pregnant
- lower abdomen cold to the touch
- infrequent or irregular periods.

If Cold is allowed to invade the Uterus it becomes difficult for a woman to conceive. Many treatments focused upon female fertility aim to warm the Uterus. The contracting energy of Cold sat within this area also causes problems with the menstrual cycle which is also often accompanied with cramps.

Marrow (Sui) and Brain (Nao) Disturbances

The most common imbalances of the Marrow and Brain are: Marrow deficiency and Brain Qi deficiency. These are discussed below.

Marrow Deficiency

Classical signs of Marrow deficiency are:

- congenital spinal conditions
- spine weakness
- poor memory
- weak mental faculties.

The Marrow grows from the Jing and so weaknesses here are usually linked to congenital disorders. Weaknesses and abnormalities of the spine are linked to a weakness in the Marrow; often, but not always, these are present from birth. Since the Marrow grows into the brain a weakness here may result in poor short term memory and a slow mind. A feeling of mental cloudiness is also possibly linked to a weakness in the Marrow. Often conditions of the Marrow are treated through strengthening the Kidneys.

Brain Qi Deficiency

Classical signs of Brain Qi deficiency are:

- lack of an information filter
- incoherent thoughts and actions.

Brain Qi deficiency is essentially a more serious manifestation of a Marrow deficiency. Weakness of the Brain's energy results in the 'filtering system' provided by the Brain being weakened; excess information comes through, resulting in signs we would normally associate with insanity.

Internal Causes of Disease: Food and Poor Lifestyle

What we eat has a direct influence upon the body. The body extracts energy from the food we eat and so the quality of our food will dictate the quality of the energy which the body derives from it. If we are to attain a high level of internal balance then we must provide our body with a high quality source of energy. The study of food according to Chinese medicine is long and complex; it is beyond the scope of this book to go into great detail concerning diet. Instead we will look at a few simple dietary concepts.

Moderation

To the ancient Daoists, too little food was as damaging as the overconsumption of food. If a person eats too little they will not receive the energy that the body requires and consequently they will become deficient in nature. Eating too much food will overstrain the Stomach and the Spleen which deal with the initial stages of processing the food; the result of this will be a build-up of Damp and Phlegm in the body which leads to the development of fat.

The theory of moderation also applies to the balance of meat and vegetables within the body. Too much meat is very bad for the body and leads to many health problems which the Western world is thankfully beginning to wake up to. Also, according to Daoism, vegetarianism is not that healthy for the body either. From a Western perspective it is possible for a vegetarian to ensure that they receive adequate proteins through close analysis of their diet but according to Daoism the Jing of the meat is different and equally essential. The energetic vibration of the Qi contained within meat provides essential elements for our body which strengthen the Blood and Qi of the body as well as strengthening the tendons and muscles. The only way to balance this out is to attain a high level in Nei Gong or Daoist alchemical practices whereby this energy is drawn directly from the environment itself. My personal experience of Daoists who are training in the classical way is that initiates still eat meat and only when they attain a certain level do they become vegetarian.

This viewpoint can often be unpopular due to the amount of people who choose to become vegetarian in modern times. I often give the following advice to my own students: if you are vegetarian for ethical reasons then remain vegetarian. Compromising your morals damages your level of internal health at the core of your soul far more than not eating meat. If, however, you choose to be vegetarian for health reasons, perhaps you should take a look at your health and ask yourself if it would benefit from you eating meat.

Obviously the quality of the meat you are eating needs to be taken into account. With modern farming methods and the chemicals and hormones which are added to our meat, organic meat is the best option although it is still far from perfect. The amount of meat eaten also needs to be carefully looked at; as guidance, eating good quality meat twice or, at most, three times a week is a healthy amount for an average adult.

What also needs taking into account is that these are only guidelines and of course everybody is different; what is good for one person may not be good for another. Whatever your view, a good deal of study into the food you consume is essential for maintaining a high level of health.

Food Qualities

The ethos of moderation also applies to the nature of the food which you eat. Too much spicy food leads to internal Heat. It particularly damages the Liver and Stomach as well as scattering the body's Qi and driving the emotions to become disturbed. Excessive consumption of cold food causes the Spleen to weaken as it does not like to be cold; it also causes the lower Jiao of the Triple Heater and the lower Dan Tien to become stagnant. Ice cream is the worst food that you can eat for the health of the Spleen, lower Jiao and lower Dan Tien.

Excessive sweet and sugary food damages the function of the Spleen which will produce Damp and Phlegm; a precursor to the body becoming fat. In the same way, too much dairy food will also lead to excessive internal Dampness developing.

Too much salty food damages the Kidneys; this is particularly important to keep in mind as many countries in Europe insist on putting excess salt on their food despite the fact that much of our food already has salt artificially added to it.

Please consult a detailed book on Chinese food therapy for more information on this subject.

Poor Lifestyle

The Daoist rule with regards to moderation also applies to our lifestyle and in particular the amount of exercise we do. If the body becomes inactive for too long it leads to internal stagnation of Qi and Blood which leads to hypo-function of the organs while too much activity is draining for our Qi levels as well as potentially damaging to the muscles and tendons.

The Western approach to exercise is often one of 'no pain no gain'. While this approach to exercise has its place it should not be applied to everything that we do. As a teacher of martial arts I find that pushing the body to its limits sometimes is good for developing stamina as well as for strengthening the will-power, but at the same time it is draining. In the Daoist arts we are trying to build ourselves up rather than break ourselves down. This mentality is important not only for our health but also for our level of internal development.

Emotional Imbalances Leading to Internal Imbalance

Emotional stillness is a prized state of being within the Daoist tradition. Emotions are seen as energetic movements born from the centre of our consciousness. These disturbances spread out from our centre through the energy body like waves on the surface of a lake. As they spread out they change the frequency of the whole energetic system. While we are not trying to rid ourselves of emotions we aim, within Daoism, to calm them and bring them under our control. In this way they do not disperse our energy and move the state of our mind and body out of balance. For those practising Daoist alchemy, stilling of the emotions is particularly important as excessive emotional activity causes the Shen energy to deplete. The spiritual treasure of Shen is built up through Daoist sitting practices with the aim of connecting to the power of Heaven and ultimately Dao. If the Shen is dispersed by excessive heightened emotional activity then the higher levels of alchemy are difficult to attain.

Table 8.1 shows the energetic and organ associations of the five emotions.

Table 8.1: The Emotions

	Excitation	Worry	Grief/Sadness	Fear	Anger
Element	Fire	Earth	Metal	Water	Wood
Movement	Expansion	Division	Contraction	Sinking	Shooting
Yin Organ	Heart	Spleen	Lungs	Kidneys	Liver
Yang Organ	Small Intestine	Stomach	Large Intestine	Bladder	Gall Bladder

An excess in any one of the five emotions in Table 8.1 may begin to damage the energy of the organ and elemental energies attached to that emotion. For example, excessive worry may begin to damage the Spleen and the Stomach leading to digestive issues while excessive anger may damage the Liver and Gall Bladder. In the same way, the energy of one of the organs being affected may also lead to the emotion associated with that organ becoming an issue. For example, if the Spleen becomes imbalanced then a person may begin to worry excessively; if the Liver's energy is disturbed it may cause a person to anger more easily.

This is because the emotion is only a manifestation of one of the five spiritual lights which move down through the energetic realm, into the physical realms where they form a bodily organ. The emotion of anger is as much Wood energy as the Liver is and so on with each of the five key emotions.

It may seem over-simplified since there are only five key emotions but you must remember that they are only categories. Many other emotions and states of mind fit into these categories. Some of these are summarised in Table 8.2.

Table 8.2: **Emotion Categories**

Excitation	Worry	Grief/Sadness	Fear	Anger
Happiness	Over-thinking	Depression	Nervousness	Frustration
Mania	Pensiveness	Melancholy	Timidity	Annoyance
	Nervousness	Loss	Terror	Self-hate
		Despair	Shock	Stress
			Insecurity	

The Emotions as Diagnostic Tools

If you are prone to one of the emotional disturbances listed above then this can be used as an external diagnostic sign that the related organ is out of balance in some way. For example, if you are prone to outbursts of manic laughter then this is clearly excitation linked to an imbalance within the energy of the Heart. If you are prone to outbursts of irrational anger then this is clearly an imbalance within the energy of the Liver.

The only exception to this is depression. This is a complex emotional disturbance which is linked to the energy of the Lungs in the table above. This is an over-simplification since depression can also be caused by a stagnation of the energy of the Liver or by weakness within the Heart's energy. Depression needs to be studied alongside other diagnostic signs and exploration of the meridian pathways to seek out imbalances.

BOX 8.1: TRANSMISSION FOR THERAPISTS

During the course of any therapeutic treatment there is an exchange of energy/information taking place. I have met many therapy practitioners who disagree with this; they have told me that under no circumstances does their particular therapy transfer energy from one person to another. I would say to this that any interaction, whether it involves contact or not, results in an exchange of energy; not just therapeutic interactions. This energetic exchange is the nature of life. Over the years I have become increasingly sensitive to the movement of energy and when observing treatments carried out by therapists I can safely say that energy is indeed moving from one person to another. Since this is the case, it is important to look at the responsibility therapists have to themselves and their patients.

When you are treating a patient then some of the information from your energy body is going to be having an effect upon them. This is reinforced by the fact that they have come to you for treatment, the balance between the two of you is not equal. Essentially the therapist is in a more powerful position; the patient is in a far more receptive and ultimately vulnerable position. The information from your energy body will very easily be passed on to them whether you wish it to or not. This places a responsibility on the therapist to ensure that they remain as healthy and as balanced as they can be. Their energy must be free-flowing and they must strive to ensure that they are in a high level of physical and emotional health as well. If not then the information passed to the patient will either be insufficient to assist them in their healing process or, worse, it will be detrimental to their health. For this reason every therapist should have some kind of health maintenance practice of their own. The practices outlined in this book would be ideal for any practitioners of energy therapies such as Qi Gong healing for example as it assists in the energetic balancing process.

It is also important to be aware of your own weaknesses, both physical and energetic. For example, if you suffer with weak lungs then you should not really be treating people with weak lungs. If you are an ethical practitioner then you should send these patients to another therapist, one with healthy lungs. This also applies to emotional issues; if you are depressed then do not treat people with depression. Some may argue that the person suffering with depression would be more empathetic towards a patient with depression so therefore they would be a better therapist but this is not taking the factor of energetic exchange into account.

Further Study

This has been an overview of the nature and causes of disease according to Daoist thought. As with any internal subject such as this, the theory can go much deeper; the information in this chapter should serve as a foundation for further study. In order to understand the reasons for the different manifestations and symptoms which come from weakening Yin and Yang aspects of the Zang Fu organs you should refer back to Chapter 7 and cross reference the Yin and Yang functions of the organs against the various imbalances which they can manifest. If you spend sufficient time doing this the energetic mysteries of the inner environment of your body can start to open up to you.

The next chapter looks at the celestial pillar, the last major area of possible imbalance which is covered in this book before practical exercises to bring about change are discussed. Remember that the theory will inform your practice, so do not be in too much of a hurry to skip past the chapters which cover the theory of the body. Be diligent and build yourself a strong foundation.

CHAPTER 9

THE CELESTIAL PILLAR

One last aspect of the human body to look at with regards to imbalance is the spine. The spine is a physical support which upholds the structure of the body; it encases the spinal cord providing protection as well as supporting the ribs which protect the organs contained within the chest. Within Daoism it also contains the spinal branch of the thrusting meridian as well as connecting to the governing meridian and the inner branches of the Bladder meridian. Due to the passageway of essential physical, energetic and spiritual substances through the body it is sometimes referred to as the celestial pillar within Daoist schools; the physical manifestation of the thoroughfare between Heaven and Earth. Figure 9.1 shows the various meridian connections to the spine.

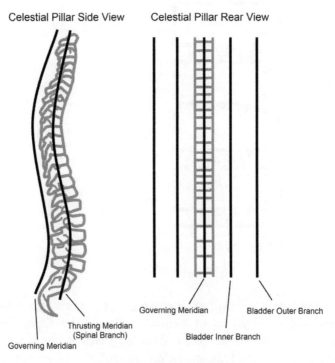

Figure 9.1: The Celestial Pillar

The spine is connected to the organs of the body on a physical level via the nervous system and energetically via the branches which run from between the vertebrae deeper into the body. These small branches also connect in to the Bladder meridian meaning that the inner posterior branch of the Bladder meridian can be used to treat not only spinal problems but also imbalances within any of the Zang Fu organs of the body.

We can use the spine within our practice to assess the health of our organs as an organ weakness will cause the vertebral space linked to that particular organ to close up. The energy within the small collateral branch of the meridian system linking the organ to the vertebral space will become deficient in Qi. This lack of energy will mean that the fluid which exists in the intervertebral disc diminishes bringing the vertebrae closer together. The result is that the muscles around this area will tighten and mobility between the vertebrae in this area will lessen or vanish completely as the vertebrae stick together. Conversely, an injury to the back which damages the vertebrae will have a detrimental effect upon the Qi which is delivered to the organs via this area of the body. Figure 9.2 summarises this process.

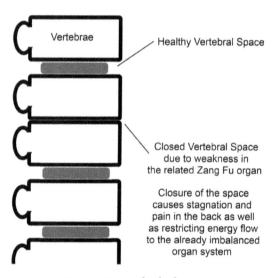

Figure 9.2: Vertebral Closure

We may not only use this understanding of the spine as a diagnostic tool but also as a method of treatment. Clearing blockages from the meridians connected to the spine and restoring energy flow here can free up mobility within the back and help to nourish the organ connected to each individual vertebra.

The Vertebral Spaces

The links between the vertebral spaces and the organs of the body are shown in Table 9.1. Please note that these are the energetic connections rather than physical via the nervous system.

Table 9.1: Spinal Connections

Vertebral Space	Connection	Associated Point
Skull – C1	Blood Supply to Head	Fengfu (GV16)
C1 – C2	Tongue	Yamen (GV15)
C2 – C3	Eyes	No associated points
C3 – C4	Ears	No associated points
C4 – C5	Vocal Cords	No associated points
C5 – C6	Pharynx	No associated points
C6 – C7	Thyroid Gland	No associated points
C7 – T1	Whole Spine	Dazhui (GV14)
T1 – T2	Middle Dan Tien	Taodao (GV13)
T2 – T3	Wind Energy*	Fengmen (BL12)
T3 – T4	Lungs	Feishu (BL13)
T4 – T5	Pericardium	Jueyinshu (BL14)
T5 – T6	Heart	Xinshu (BL15)
T6 – T7	Governing Meridian	Dushu (BL16)
T7 – T8	Diaphragm	Geshu (BL17)
T8 – T9	Pancreas	Extra point between BL17 and BL18
T9 – T10	Liver	Ganshu (BL18)
T10 – T11	Gall Bladder	Danshu (BL19)
T11 – T12	Spleen	Pishu (BL20)
T12 – L1	Stomach	Weishu (BL21)
L1 – L2	Triple Heater	Sanjiaoshu (BL22)
L2 – L3	Kidneys	Shenshu (BL23)
L3 – L4	Lower Dan Tien	Qihaishu (BL24)
L4 – L5	Large Intestines	Dachangshu (BL25)
L5 – Sacrum	Sexual Organs	Guanyuanshu (BL26)

* Wind Energy. This point is actually linked closely to the muscles of the neck and upper back but it is usually understood within Daoist medicinal practices to be a point utilised in the expelling of external Wind environmental energy.

Table 9.1 shows the spaces that exist between the 24 moveable vertebrae of the spine as well as between the skull and the top of the sacrum. The nine fused bones of the sacrum and coccyx also have connections to the rest of the body but they are very difficult to work with through the practices outlined within this book; for this reason they are not included. The above table gives a list of points and vertebral spaces that may be readily worked with using the techniques in this and following chapters.

Along with the connecting part of the body that relates to each vertebral space is the associated meridian point which is generally understood to be the most effective point for nourishing any weaknesses in this area. Some of the vertebral spaces do not have associated points but this is not important. For those who are not so familiar with the structure of the spine, Figure 9.3 shows the vertebrae of the spine.

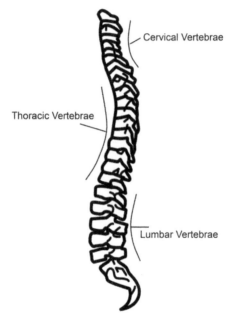

Figure 9.3: The Spine

I would urge all practitioners of any Daoist arts to become familiar with the spine and its energetic connections as they impact upon every area of Daoist study to some degree. A great many people also suffer with back problems and understanding the connection between the spine and the energy system can help move towards healing the back.

The Spinal Curves

It should be noted here that the spine is supposed to have a smooth and healthy curvature to it. This is how the spine is designed. There are many Qi Gong practices which aim to straighten the spine; the belief is that the spine is able to transfer much more energy along its length if the spine is straightened out. This is not true. Daoist practices always aim to adhere to the natural state of things; to remove the 'S' curve from the spine is to go against what it natural and should not be done. This inhibits the flow of energy rather than strengthens it and generates tension in the body; tension which will later turn into stagnation, pain and illness. Any work to address a person's posture should take the healthy, natural curved shape of the spine into account.

Assessing the Health of the Celestial Pillar

With the increase in popularity of alternative therapists such as chiropractors many people are already aware of any issues in their spine. Many students who come to me with health problems are also aware of exactly which vertebrae are connected to the issue. This obviously makes assessment of the spine easy providing that the assessment of the spine has been accurate. If the state of the spine is unknown then we need to carry out the following procedure to ascertain for ourselves exactly where the problems are located.

Sit in one of the positions shown in Figure 9.4 with your spine erect and your head suspended. Relax but do not allow your body to slump down.

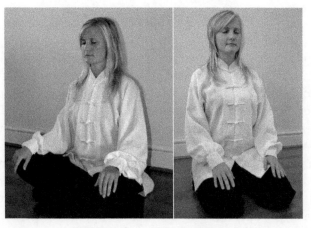

Figure 9.4: Floor Sitting Postures

If this is uncomfortable for you then sit upright in a chair but be aware that this is not as effective a posture for the practice.

Connect with your spine in the same way that you would with any of the meridians of the arms and legs. Essentially it is actually several meridians you are connecting with. It is the governing meridian which runs down the length of the middle of your back as well as the Jiaji channels which run close to the edge of your spine. The Jiaji channels in turn connect in to the Bladder meridians and can, for the purposes of this training, be thought of as transports of information between the spine and the inner Bladder branch. These channels are shown in Figure 9.5.

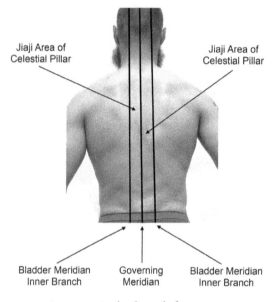

Figure 9.5: Back Channels for Assessment

You should by now be able to tune into the energy body with relative ease so you should not need a specific entrance point for the Yi. Instead just bring your mind in to gently focus upon the energy which runs along the length of the entire spine. Relax, continue to breathe deeply and let your awareness remain gently listening to the spine. It will not take too long before you are able to get a feeling for the energy of the spine.

The spine's energy tends to be less distinct in nature than the meridians you have contacted previously. Its edges are less defined because of the fact that you are assessing a few different energetic pathways at the same time. Once you have made contact with the spine's energy it is time to begin getting a feel for its quality. Look for the following characteristics:

- If the lumbar area of the spine feels tight, weak and in pain then this is usually an indicator of the Kidneys' energy being weak. Remember that an internal branch of the Kidney meridian runs through the lower back and so deficiency in either the Kidneys' Yin or Yang aspect will deplete the Qi running through the lumbar region.

- If the lumbar spine has sensations of Cold, Damp or Wind as well as tightness and pain then this is usually due to the presence of one of the environmental energies rather than a Kidney deficiency although there could also be both conditions.

- The length of the entire spine can also be checked for invading environmental energies as these may have invaded the Bladder or governing meridian and been transported into the spine.

Once you have ruled out general conditions like those listed above it is time to begin looking at individual vertebral spaces. Begin by placing your awareness on the lower spine at the point where it connects in to the sacrum. Let it hover here for a while and ensure that you still have a strong connection with the energy of the spine.

Gradually begin to run your awareness up the length of the spine near the surface of the body. Your awareness will be able to focus not only on the vertebral spaces directly on the posterior midline but also on the areas directly adjacent to the spine as shown in Figure 9.6.

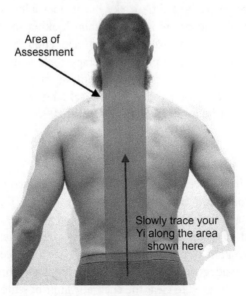

Figure 9.6: Vertebral Assessment

Move your awareness up the length of the spine taking time to examine each part of the back in detail. Hesitate the awareness every few centimetres and wait to see what information is sent to your brain for processing. If there is a blockage within the spine you will find that an area is painful. This pain can vary from being a dull ache (indicating deficiency) or a sharp pain (indicating stagnation). In many cases this pain will present itself very quickly, blockages in the spine tend to be easy to find and pretty uncomfortable.

It is unlikely, at first, that you will be able to differentiate between the individual vertebrae as your mind moves across them. You may well discover a painful area but not be able to find out which exact intervertebral space is related to that pain. The only way around this is to ask a friend to assist you in the process. Connect with the energy of the spine and then ask your friend to assist by lightly placing their finger on your back. Direct them to the area of pain and get them to mark it with a pen. Do this for all of the areas you find on your back that have abnormal sensations.

From here it is simply a case of getting your friend to run their hands along the length of your spine feeling each vertebrae. If they count from the bottom of the spine and work their way up they should be able to ascertain exactly with which vertebrae the stagnation is located. The five lumbar vertebrae are much larger while the thoracic vertebrae make up the rest of your back. The cervical vertebrae make up your neck.

This process may be a little tricky but it does allow you to gain an extra piece of diagnostic information when looking to understand the nature of your own imbalance. If you are lucky enough to have a friend who practises some kind of physical therapy such as massage then this person is likely to be very accurate in identifying the vertebrae for you.

Figure 9.7 shows some useful anatomical landmarks which can help locate the areas of imbalance you have identified.

Physical Injuries

A book on imbalances of the body would be incomplete without including information on physical injuries sustained through trauma. Musculoskeletal injuries are very common and most people who have been engaged in physically active pastimes will, at some point, have sustained some kind of physical injury. While the practices in this book are obviously inadequate for on the spot treatment of breaks, cuts and bruises they can be used to clear the energetic imprint which is always left behind by these kinds of injury.

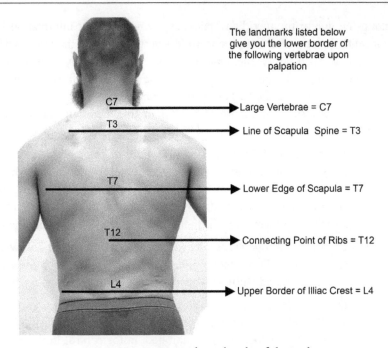

The landmarks listed below
give you the lower border of
the following vertebrae upon
palpation

C7 ▶Large Vertebrae = C7

T3 ▶ Line of Scapula Spine = T3

T7 ▶ Lower Edge of Scapula = T7

T12 ▶ Connecting Point of Ribs = T12

L4 ▶ Upper Border of Illiac Crest = L4

Figure 9.7: Anatomical Landmarks of the Back

When an injury is first sustained there will be obvious physical damage to the area. As well as this there will be a major disruption to the flow of Qi through the injury site. This information will usually stay in place long after the injury has been corrected which may in turn lead to further pain at the site or internal imbalance if the Qi moves deeper into the energy body. It is true for many conditions treated by practitioners of Chinese medicine that they may be rooted in past physical trauma. For example a physical injury which runs along the length of the Lung meridian may begin to cause a weakness in the energy of the Lungs even though this meridian runs along the length of the arm.

When working with past physical injuries you need to first assess the nature of the energetic imprint which has been left behind. The process is not so different from moving your Yi along the line of the meridian pathways to look for imbalances, blockages and so forth.

First, begin to trace your mind along any meridians which run through the site of the injury. It may be that the injury was very specific and only one meridian will need to be examined or it may be that several meridians were involved. Access them and trace your awareness along them as described previously. The first task is ascertaining which of the meridians have been affected and how far the imbalance has spread along the line of the meridians' pathway. Remember that information is transmitted along their length and so it is very likely that the injury will have left a much larger energetic imbalance than you may expect. For example, an injury to the Lung meridian at the area of the elbow may well spread right down to the length of the thumb.

When assessing the nature of the Qi in this meridian you should look for:

- *Wind Heat and Wind Cold:* Wind Heat can often be left behind by physical trauma. It usually means that the energy of the meridian in this area has become deficient, allowing external Wind to enter the body here. If left for long periods of time it can lead to arthritic type symptoms further along the length of the meridian.

- *Cold:* This pathogen is usually left after old joint injuries. This will prevent energy from moving past this point leading to tightness of the joints and stiffness which is generally worse on cold days.

- *Damp:* If Damp appears at an old injury site then the area will usually feel heavy. It is also common for people with this kind of localised imbalance to have inhibited motor control in this area of the body. Like Wind type imbalances, Damp can often lead to arthritic type conditions further along the length of the meridian. The pain and tightness usually gets worse in damp weather.

- *Heat:* An easily aggravated injury site will often leave Heat behind. This is very common in injuries which directly affected the muscles of the body. It is common for people with this kind of old injury to feel annoyed when they re-experience pain in this area.

- *Stagnant Qi:* Stagnant Qi is almost a certainty in the case of past physical injury. It is usually accompanied by one of the other energetic imbalances described here.

- *Qi Deficiency:* If there is a deficiency of energy to this area then the muscles in the area will be weakened resulting in a great reduction of strength and mobility of the body.

- *Blood Stasis:* If the information at an old injury site leads to Blood stagnating here then there will usually be sharp stabbing pains which can last for many years, particularly if the injury site is not mobilised sufficiently.

Any of these imbalances can be left behind by physical trauma. Ascertaining the type of imbalance can help to clear it from the body and in some cases give further information as to the cause of internal imbalances you may have. The sensation experienced by these imbalances is the same as described in Chapter 6 of this book.

When assessing the nature of the energy left behind by a past injury it is useful to compare it to the other side of the body. It is a fairly safe assumption that the energy on the uninjured side of the body is healthier than the side that has been damaged. If you are unfortunate enough to have sustained the same injury on both sides of the body at the same time then obviously this is not so easy.

Many people's lives are plagued with discomfort from old injuries. The energetic imbalances left behind by musculoskeletal injuries can last for the rest of a person's life if exercises are not carried out to clear the imbalances. You should spend a great deal of time connecting to the meridians in the site of old injuries and shifting the imbalanced energy here. To do this access the nearest exit point for this meridian. These points are given in Table 9.2.

It is worth keeping this practice up for some time. Look for clear signs of progress including enhanced flexibility, a softening of the area and a reduction in pain. Be aware that the time required to achieve results in this process can vary a great deal depending upon how long ago you sustained the injury. Obviously a long running imbalance resulting from an injury sustained long ago will take longer to work with than injury only a year or so old. Throughout this process keep returning to the process of assessing the energy at the injury site to see if imbalances are beginning to clear. You could also consider seeing a skilled acupuncturist a few times to assist in the process of shifting any stagnant Qi in the area. There is an important point used in the treatment of any kind of physical injury: Gall Bladder 34 (Yanglingquan). This point can be used to rejuvenate the Qi and Jing at any injury site in the body. Any session working with an old injury should also include a few minutes of activation of this point. For more detailed information on this point please see the point commentaries in Chapter 11.

Table 9.2: Exit Points for Meridian Blockages

Meridian Affected by Injury	Easiest Exit Point
Heart Meridian	Heart 9 – Shaochong
Small Intestine Meridian	Small Intestine 1 – Shaoze
Pericardium Meridian	Pericardium 9 – Zhongchong
Triple Heater Meridian	Triple Heater 1 – Guanchong
Spleen Meridian	Spleen 1 – Yinbai
Stomach Meridian	Stomach 45 – Lidui
Lung Meridian	Lung 11 – Shaoshang
Large Intestine Meridian	Large Intestine 1 – Shangyang
Kidney Meridian	Kidney 1 – Yongquan
Bladder Meridian	Bladder 64 – Jingu
Liver Meridian	Liver 1 – Dadun
Gall Bladder Meridian	Gall Bladder 44 – Zuqiaoyin

CHAPTER 10

BUILDING A PICTURE

The final stage in creating an assessment of your own internal environment is putting all of the information you have gathered together into one big picture. This involves looking at the information you have gained from internal observation of the meridians as well as information drawn from external observations. Once this picture has been put together you may begin to form a strategy for changing the nature of this environment to move yourself closer to a state of balance.

By now you should have some information drawn from your own internal exploration. It is important that this information is very recent as the human energy system is in a state of constant flux; readings taken a few weeks ago may have changed considerably. While chronic imbalances will most likely still be present, any environmental energies flowing through the meridians will certainly have shifted to some degree. This is the nature of energy, it is never constant. This means that although you may manage to clear a section of your meridians, freeing up energy flow, you must return to this practice regularly to keep yourself healthy and your Qi flowing smoothly. In this way, the practices in this book can be added to your training routine as a kind of energetic overhaul which you do every now and then. Remember that it is also a key point of this book that the practices should help lead you towards gaining a strong experiential understanding of the energy body. There is a great deal of learning to be had from going through the processes in this book even if no major imbalances are discovered. Understanding the shifting energies of the microcosm of your meridian system forms the foundation for understanding the shifting energies of the macrocosm and how you relate to it.

Your Self-Analysis

Your personal analysis of your own energy system is made up from several pieces of information. These pieces of information are the result of asking yourself several questions; these questions are summarised here:

1. *Were there any major elemental imbalances present within your energy system?* Is it clear from the signs outlined in Chapter 2 that you have a tendency towards any one of the five elemental energies? All people have different percentages of the elements, this is quite normal. It only becomes a problem when one of the elements is so out of balance that it is creating negative effects upon the mind and body. Rebalancing the five elements should be the first step in your practice and so you should use the Wu Xing Qi Gong as described in Chapter 2 to work with these energies. This process can take some time and you will never completely rebalance the five elements; you should just aim to 'take the edge off' your key imbalance. If you have excessive signs of Wood, for example, then you should aim to practise the Wu Xing Qi Gong until this elemental excess is not so prominent.

2. *Do you have a tendency towards the pathogenic manifestation of any of the six environmental energies?* Does your body have a tendency towards any of the six environmental energies? Perhaps you have been over-exposed to one of these types of Qi within the environment or perhaps your own energy system has produced the internal manifestation of these energies due to an imbalance. Make a note of any obvious tendency towards one of the six environmental energies discussed in Chapter 4. We will see how to clear these pathogens in this chapter.

3. *Were there any imbalances present within any of the meridian pathways?* Did you discover any blockages or imbalances present within any of the meridians you explored? It is unlikely that all of your meridian pathways were completely free of imbalances. Make a note of any imbalances present within any of the meridians as discussed in Chapter 6. If you had a tendency towards any one particular type of imbalance then this is an important indicator.

4. *Do the external signs show you have an imbalance within any of the organs of the body?* Do you have any clear externally manifested signs of Zang Fu weakness as described in Chapter 8. This is nothing to worry about; everybody has a tendency towards one or more Zang Fu organs being out of balance.

5. *Do you have any physical injuries which need rebalancing?* Do you any physical imbalances as outlined in the previous chapter?

Putting it all Together

You should now have a list of imbalances discovered through the exploration of your own internal energy system. It is time to begin putting it all together. Are there are patterns forming? It is highly unlikely that all of your symptoms are completely unrelated; you should be able to understand their relationship to see if there are any key themes running through your own energy system.

Ask yourself the following questions:

- Does your elemental imbalance match any organs which may be related to it? Does this elemental imbalance have any relationship to key meridians which were particularly blocked?

- Did any of the external environmental energies match the related organs or six divisional meridians which are usually associated with that pathogen?

- Did any meridians which were particularly blocked match the Zang Fu organs which were out of balance? Did this also match your elemental imbalance?

- Did any imbalances within the meridians or Zang Fu organs match tendencies towards strong emotional imbalances you may have?

- Do any physical pains and injuries radiate down the length of meridians which relate to an organ you also have a clear weakness within?

Asking yourself these questions should help you to bring together all of the information to generate a good picture of any energetic tendencies you may have. It may be wise to write down these imbalances; keep a kind of diary of imbalances you have found. Over time, practising these methods should start to give you an interesting idea of how energy is shifting within you. It is often interesting to see how these energetic imbalances are related to seasonal changes, times of the day and phases of the moon. Understanding these patterns can also help towards understanding how you relate to the wider environment.

A Case Example

Person A has carried out the entire process within this book. He has studied the methodologies outlined here for a few months and managed to reach the stage of connecting to and understanding the information contained within the meridians' pathways. Person A has a stressful job which places a lot of pressure upon him. He has tight joints which cause him to ache a great deal and he has been diagnosed by Western doctors as having arthritis in his right foot. He is prone to feelings of frustration and anger which is often vented on his work colleagues and family members.

He ascertained that he clearly had a tendency towards a Wood elemental imbalance and so, in the early stages of his practice, began working on the Wu Xing Qi Gong with an aim to subdue the Wood elemental energy. He practised all five exercises every morning with an emphasis on the Metal elemental exercise which helps to control Wood via the Ke cycle of the five element theory. Over the space of a few weeks person A found that he was less stressed at work; he was less prone to feelings of anger being directed at the people around him. He began to adopt these exercises at home as well prior to sleeping and continued to find that they had a soothing effect upon his Wood elemental aspect.

Feeling ready to move on, person A began to look at the six environmental energy signs. He saw that he disliked being in hot environments; he always felt hot inside anyway so always tried to be in cool rooms. At work he would always open the windows and put a fan on. He was also prone to being thirsty a lot; no matter how much water he drank he was still thirsty. From this he decided that he had a tendency towards the environmental energy of Heat. It was unclear to him at this point whether or not this Heat was internal or external in origin.

Over time person A began successfully to connect with his meridians via the Yuan source point and spent a few weeks connecting with the various pathways of his energy system. Upon searching for imbalances he found that there was an excess of Heat signs in his Heart meridian and Liver meridian; the Heat in the Liver meridian was particularly strong around the area of his foot where he had previously identified arthritis. As well as Heat signs in the meridians there were several areas which felt blocked; these were spread around different meridians and seemed to have no particular pattern. Upon further exploration of the area of his foot he discovered that the Liver meridian also contained Damp blockages which were present mostly around the area of his foot.

Now that he had explored the internal energy system, Person A began to look at the external signs which may help indicate organ imbalances. When particularly stressed at work he had previously had temporal headaches which sometimes led to dizziness; this combined with his angry emotional state indicated the diagnosis of 'Liver Yang rising'.

Person A now had clear information on the state of his energy body. All of the signs indicated internal Heat, excessive Wood energy which manifested in Liver Yang rising as well as Damp and Heat blocking the Liver meridian in the area of his foot. The rebalancing strategy selected from the next section of this chapter would aim to address these issues.

Conclusion

This is the process of identifying your own internal imbalance. Please note that internal imbalance is very different from 'disease'. Everybody has a tendency towards an energetic imbalance of some kind so it is nothing to be concerned about. Energetic imbalances can be redressed so it is an empowering stage to be at once you have identified the state of your energy body.

Initiating Change

The process of initiating change is fairly simple. In order to change the nature of the energy body we need to access it in the same way that we previously accessed the meridian system; we use the meridian points to translate the frequency of our awareness and access the energy body. Unlike before, where we only observed the nature of our internal environment, we now begin to change it using our intention. This is a practice which sits between Qi Gong and meditation; it the foundation of Daoist internal health exercises.

Along the meridian pathways lay the meridian points. Each of these not only serves as a contact point between the internal energy system and the external environment but also as a way to change the nature of the Qi within our body. Through connecting our awareness to the correct points we are able to activate the element of our energy body related to that point; this begins to change the intricate balance of energies within us. Through developing an understanding of these points and their transformational nature we are given an easy and efficient way to take charge of our own health, an aspect of life which people often seem resigned to place in the hands of others.

The first thing we must learn is how to activate a meridian point so that it may begin to change the nature of our Qi. For this process I suggest you use Zusanli (ST36), a commonly used point. The reason I suggest using this point is that it will not have a detrimental effect upon any internal condition which you may have identified. Some points in the body can cause a problem to become worse; for example, a point which takes Heat out of the body will not be a good point to select in people with excess internal Cold. Zusanli (ST36) is a point which has a nourishing effect upon the body's Qi and Blood; it is beneficial no matter what internal imbalances you may have. Figure 10.1 shows the location of Zusanli (ST36).

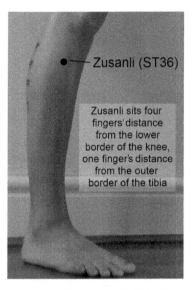

Zusanli (ST36)

Zusanli sits four
fingers' distance
from the lower
border of the knee,
one finger's distance
from the outer
border of the tibia

Figure 10.1: Zusanli (ST36)

Locate the point physically first. Follow the guidelines in Figure 10.1 and
you should find a small depression in the leg where the point is located.
Massage the point with your thumb to ensure that you are totally clear on
the location. This is a key point on the Stomach meridian which is part
of the Yang Ming divisional aspect of the body. As the Yang Ming aspect
has an abundance of both Qi and Blood, this point will help to nourish
the Qi and Blood of the body.

Once you are familiar with the location of the point, stand in the Zhan
Zhuang position you have used previously. This is shown in Figure 5.8.

This is the most effective position to ensure that the energy of the
body can flow freely but if you find this difficult then you can experiment
with connecting with the point while lying on your back. While this
point is not so efficient with regards to Qi flow it may be easier for
beginners who have difficulty relaxing the muscles of their legs while in
standing postures.

Bring your awareness (Yi) down to the point as if you were going to
access the Stomach meridian through it. You should aim to bring your
mind to the point on both legs at the same time since the meridians
are bilateral. It is quite likely that the Stomach meridian will unfold for
you as your awareness will be used to this process by now. Just ignore
the line of the Stomach meridian; while it does not matter if you have
connected with it, you do not want your awareness to begin following

the meridian's pathway. You need to keep your awareness on the point of Zusanli (ST36).

Activating the Points

The actions of meridian points can be activated in several different ways. A beginner massage therapist may press on the point which will stimulate it; this will activate the point to a very small degree and the effects will not last very long. A low level acupuncturist will simply place a needle into the point which will cause activation stronger than from a massage but it will still be fairly weak and temporary. The most skilled massage therapists, acupuncturists and so forth will combine their therapeutic techniques with their intention. The Yi must travel down the massage therapist's hands or fingers into the point to ensure full activation of the point. A skilled acupuncturist will send their intention through the length of the needle they have inserted into the point to fully activate the points they are using in their treatment; without this part of the treatment the effects will be greatly lessened. Sadly, the vast majority of modern Chinese medicine practitioners do not even accept the possibility of this process and so Chinese medicine has been greatly weakened. It is for this reason that Qi Gong exercises are an essential part of any Chinese medical practitioner's training; without Qi Gong, practitioners of therapies such as acupuncture will never progress past a shallow level of skill.

Within the techniques outlined within this book we are solely going to be using our awareness. We are bypassing the physical therapeutic technique and directing our mind straight into the required meridian points. This should be fairly easy to do as we are working with our own energy system; it takes considerably more practice to repeat these techniques on another person's energy system.

Activating a meridian point is much like gently blowing on the dying embers of a fire to ignite them to flame once more. Through a combination of our breath and awareness we cause the information stored within the Qi of a point to expand. This will activate the point causing its transformative properties to take effect. Figure 10.2 summarises this concept.

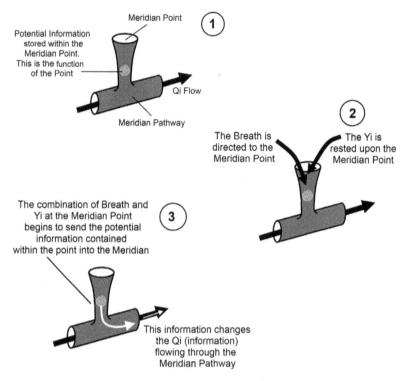

Figure 10.2: Activating a Meridian Point

It is through this process of studying and activating the meridian points of the body that the ancient Daoists devised their intricate system of meridian based medicine.

Keep your awareness on Zusanli (ST36) as you begin to 'breathe' into the point. Your Yi will lead the Qi as before. It is now that you begin to change your breathing for the first time. We are now aiming to stimulate the point rather than just connecting with it and listening to what is taking place. Put a little more emphasis into the exhalation than before; you should direct more force into your out-breath. Note that this increase in force is extremely slight. Think how much force you have to use when blowing the dying embers of a fire, it is very slight indeed. Your breathing should be in and out through the nose, keep your mouth lightly closed throughout this process. Keep with this process for a while. The extra emphasis on the exhalation coupled with the placement of your Yi will begin to stimulate more Qi to be led through the body to the meridian point.

After some time you will begin to become aware of a growing pressure in the area of Zusanli (ST36). This pressure will begin to become clearer until the point feels warm and starts to tingle. Keep with this process and observe what is taking place as you continue to lead your breath and Qi to this area. This warmth will then begin to move outwards into the Stomach meridian; once this happens, you have managed to activate the meridian point meaning that its therapeutic function has been engaged.

Keep up the practice for at least ten minutes once you have reached this stage. With practice the sensation will become stronger and begin to move out into the whole of the meridian. If the Qi and Blood are stimulated to a high degree you will also find that the feeling of warmth and tingling spreads out into the rest of your body. This is a very nourishing practice which has great benefit to your general well-being.

Do not worry if this stage in your practice is difficult; it can take time. Just as with learning to connect with the meridians, it can take practice and perseverance. Stick with it though and before long you will have managed to activate your first meridian point using only your intention and breath. This is an important step as it means that you now have an effective way to adjust the health of your body at its energetic root. This root is the most effective place to change if you wish to bring lasting balance to the whole of your mind-body system.

As stated above, Zusanli (ST36) is a good meridian point to practise on due to its safe and nourishing effect upon the Qi and Blood of the body. Even if you discover very little in the way of internal imbalance, this is still an effective point to work with as everybody could do with a boost to their Qi every now and then.

Practise regularly until you are able to contact and activate this point quickly and easily. From here you can begin to activate further points on the body according to your own personal needs.

Selecting the Points

There are many meridian points spread across the surface of the body. They are connected to all parts of the meridian system and have innumerable therapeutic functions which can be tapped into in the same way as when using Zusanli (ST36). These points, however, should not be chosen at random for your practice. The state of your internal energy system is held in delicate balance. The powers of Yin and Yang are intermixing to different degrees within you resulting in your personal state of being. The activation of various points will begin to change this balance and you should be aware that you need to move your internal environment towards a state of central equilibrium rather than further away from this point. While being further from equilibrium this will not cause you serious harm, it is counterproductive to your own personal development and will move you further away from building the foundation required for further spiritual development.

When listing points in the next chapter I have outlined not only their location and therapeutic functions but also any contra-indications to their use. These are contra-indications which differ from those normally indicated within contemporary Chinese medicine; they are aimed at those carrying out Daoist internal exercise as outlined in this book.

I have also indicated what internal imbalance the point is useful for as well as helpful combinations if there are any that apply. I have aimed the point descriptions at non-Chinese medical practitioners so the information may differ from the information you will commonly find in acupuncture textbooks.

A Practice Session

Once you have ascertained the nature of your own imbalance you should begin to familiarise yourself with all of the points I have listed in the next chapter. Make sure you have an overview of the various points so that you can select them effectively. Putting together your own personal prescription of points is an art form, not an exact science. It may take a bit of experimentation to discover which points are most effective for you. If you find that one point is particularly effective then you may want to focus more on this point's activation than others you have selected.

During one practice session you should aim to select around three or four points. The majority of these are bilateral as the meridians are reflected on both sides of the body so you will obviously aim to be focusing on both these points at the same time. Do not worry too much which order you focus upon the points although as a general rule of thumb you start at the top of the head and work down towards the feet. Points on the governing and conception meridians are not bilateral as they sit on the anterior and posterior midline.

Once you have selected your points you should decide what posture you are going to use. You have three options: standing in Zhan Zhuang, sitting cross legged or lying down as shown in Figure 10.3.

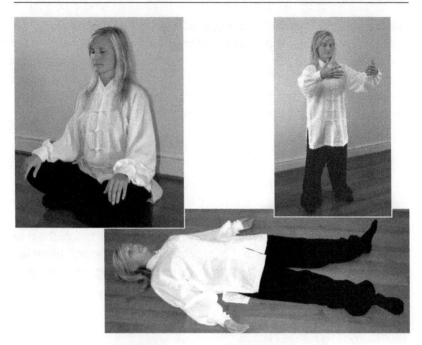

Figure 10.3: Point Activation Postures

There are different benefits to each of these three postures which are outlined below. These should be taken into account when selecting your practice posture.

Zhan Zhuang

This posture enables you to access all of the points very effectively as it is the prime posture for effective energy flow through the body. The difficulty with this posture is that beginners may be too tense in this position to maintain it long enough for effective practice. It will also be ineffective if your posture is incorrect. This can easily be remedied by going to a Qi Gong teacher whom you trust in the local area. The vast majority of Qi Gong teachers will be familiar with this posture and so should be able to correct you.

Sitting Cross Legged

This position allows for good contact with the Earth because of your near vicinity to the floor. The upright positioning of the spine coupled with the strong Earth contact means that it is easier to open the thrusting meridian in the posture. The result of this is that points along the governing meridian, conception meridian and those located on the head are easier to activate. The problems with this posture come from the fact that you will find it difficult, but not impossible, to work with points located on the legs. Beginners will also have the problem of tension in the back and legs making practice painful and difficult.

Lying Down

Lying on your back is the least effective position out of the three but has the advantage of enabling the whole body to easily relax. This may be a good starting posture for those new to Daoist internal practices. It is also useful for those who wish to practise when they go to bed before they fall asleep. Note though that once the Qi begins to move, you will likely fall asleep due to the calming effects that the energy moving has upon you; this may cut your practice short.

Combining Postures

It is fine to combine postures in one practice session. You may wish to start sitting cross legged on the floor while you work with points on the head and body before standing up into Zhan Zhuang so that you may work on points located on the legs. Just ensure that the change between postures is carried out slowly and smoothly so that you remain calm throughout your practice.

Activate each of the points you have selected. With practice you will know when they have activated but for those starting out in this practice I have indicated within the description for each point what the sensation for Qi activation in this area is most likely to feel like; this information is drawn from my own personal experience and that of my students.

When you have worked through all of the points and wish to conclude your practice you should follow your breathing for a minute before walking briskly around for a few minutes. You may even wish to run through the Wu Xing Qi Gong afterwards as they will complement your training.

CHAPTER 11

MERIDIAN POINTS

What follows now is a discussion of the location, therapeutic functions, contra-indications and common uses of key points on the body. There are a great deal more points on the body than are covered in this chapter. I have only included key meridian points relevant to the practices outlined within this book. I have also included only those that are practical for use in your training. Though some points are very useful, they are also very difficult to locate on your own so I have omitted them from these lists.

Please familiarise yourself with all of the points before embarking on training to adjust your internal climate to ensure that you are able to select points for activation effectively. After the points have been described I have included tables of point categories for ease of selection. Please note that some of the information in this chapter may differ from the contemporary Chinese medicine understanding of the meridian points.

I have also only included meridian points which are safe to use. There are many others which can be accessed with the methods outlined in this book; many of them are very powerful but also carry some element of risk. I would recommend that you only use the points listed in this chapter as some of the others can be detrimental to your health if used in the wrong way. The use of these points requires extensive personal instruction.

For each meridian point I have given the standard Chinese name in Pinyin followed by the commonly understood numerical system used by Western acupuncturists.

Note that the location descriptions have been kept deliberately simple to follow. For those who wish to have more detailed location descriptions I would recommend using: *A Manual of Acupuncture* by Peter Deadman (2007) which is produced by the Journal of Chinese Medicine Publications.

Useful Points on the Heart Meridian

Useful points along the pathway of the Heart meridian include: Jiquan (HE1), Shaohai (HE3), Lingdao (HE4), Shenmen (HE7) and Shaochong (HE9). These points are shown on the diagram of the Heart meridian in Figure 11.1.

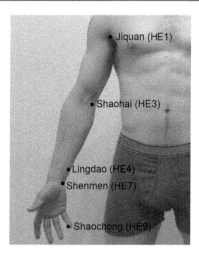

Figure 11.1: Heart Meridian Points

Jiquan (Heart 1) – 'Ultimate Spring' – 極泉

This point is the external origin of the Heart meridian. It is located in the centre of the axilla (the armpit). Put your fingers into the deepest part of the armpit and you will feel a tender point where Jiquan is located.

Therapeutic Functions: Jiquan can be accessed to regulate any imbalances in the energy of the Heart. These imbalances may be within the Heart's energetic functions or within the Shen which resides within the emptiness at the centre of the Heart. This point also connects in to the middle Dan Tien meaning that it is particularly useful for regulating the emotions.

Qi Sensation: This point spreads warmth around the area of the armpit when it is activated. This warmth often spreads into the area of the chest around the physical organ of the Heart.

Contra-Indications: None.

Shaohai (Heart 3) – 'Small Sea' – 少海

With the arm flexed, this point can be found at the tender spot situated at the medial end of the elbow crease.

Therapeutic Functions: Shaohai has a cooling effect upon the Heart and so should be used in cases of excess Heat caused by emotional disturbance as well as signs linked to Heart Fire. It can also be used for emotional agitation and manic behaviour which is often linked to the Shen being disturbed by Heat in the Heart.

Qi Sensation: When activated, this point begins to tingle. This tingling sensation then begins to move along the length of the meridian towards the hand as it clears the Heat vibrational information from the area of the Heart.

Contra-Indications: Do not use in any conditions where the Heart's energy is deficient.

Lingdao (Heart 4) – 'Spiritual Path' – 靈道

Lingdao is situated on the inside of the wrist. From Shenmen (HE7) this point is two fingers' breadth down the wrist towards the elbow. It is sat on the radial side of the flexor tendon.

Therapeutic Functions: The name of the point suggests that it helps the spirit of the Heart find its way back to the correct path. Therapeutically it can be used for any Heart imbalance, especially those of a deficient nature.

Qi Sensation: When activated, this point often feels as if there is pressure building in the area. It is sometimes described as feeling as though somebody is pressing on the point with their finger. This pressure begins to move along the line of the meridian as the information is passed into the meridian system.

Contra-Indications: None.

Shenmen (Heart 7) – 'Gate of the Spirit' – 神門

Shenmen is located on the inside of the wrist. It is sat on the wrist crease to the radial side of the flexor tendon. To locate it you can slide your finger down off of the pisiform bone of the hand into the depression on the wrist crease.

Therapeutic Functions: This point is the Yuan source point of the Heart meridian meaning that it has a strong connection with the outside energy. It is also the point you most likely used to access the Heart meridian in your earlier practices. It can be used for all spiritual and emotional imbalances related to the energy of the Heart. Since all emotions are to some degree linked to the Heart you may activate this point for a wide variety of reasons. It is one of the most commonly used points within Chinese medicine when treating the psyche. It should be noted though that it should not be used on those with depression.

Qi Sensation: When this point is observed, as in your earlier practices, it enabled you to make contact with the length of the meridian but now you are adding the power of your Qi via the breathing method outlined in the previous chapter. This will cause the point to fully activate which results in a comforting warmth which spreads out across the length of the meridian. You will usually also notice that your mind becomes very still when this point is activated as the emptiness at the centre of your Heart is directly contacted. It literally opens the 'Gate of the Spirit' so that your Shen may re-enter the Heart.

Contra-Indications: This point should not be activated if you suffer with any form of depression. This is due to the fact that this point is also the sedation point of the Heart according to Daoist thought. Sedating the Heart is fine unless a person is depressed. The sedated Heart energy will not be able to control Metal (via the five element control cycle) meaning that any depression linked to a Metal imbalance may worsen.

Shaochong (Heart 9) – 'Small Surge' – 少沖

Shaochong is situated on the inside corner of the little finger nail. If you drew a line connecting the base of the nail and the inside border of the nail then the connecting point would be Shaochong.

Therapeutic Functions: Shaochong can be used with these practices to dredge the length of the Heart meridian. It can help to clear any blockages or imbalances which you discovered in your examination of the Heart meridian pathway.

Qi Sensation: When activated it will feel as though there is a warm breeze blowing out of the end of your little finger. It is a very strange sensation at first but a very pleasant one. As the breeze continues you may feel sensations of energy moving out of the body via the length of the Heart meridian.

Contra-Indications: None.

Useful Points on the Small Intestine Meridian

Useful points along the pathway of the Small Intestine meridian include: Shaoze (SI1), Houxi (SI3), Wangu (SI4), Jianzhen (SI9), Tianchuang (SI16) and Tinggong (SI19). These points are shown on the diagram of the Small Intestine meridian in Figure 11.2.

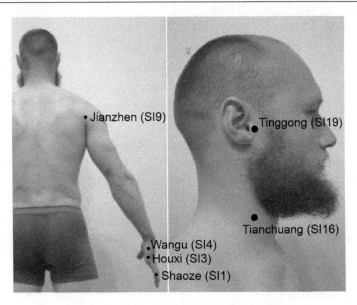

Figure 11.2: Small Intestine Meridian Points

Shaoze (Small Intestine 1) – 'Small Marsh' – 少澤

This is the start point of the external branch of the Small Intestine meridian. It is located at the outer corner of the little finger nail at the point where the outer border and the base of the nail would intersect if two lines were drawn.

Therapeutic Functions: Shaoze can be used to dredge the length of the Small Intestine meridian of any blockages or imbalances. Even though the meridian flows away from the hand towards the torso, activating this point will cause pathogens to exit the finger. It can be thought of as much like opening the stopper on the top of a container.

Qi Sensation: When activated it will feel as though there is a warm breeze blowing out of the end of your little finger. It is a very strange sensation at first but a very pleasant one. As the breeze continues you may feel sensations of energy moving out of the body via the length of the Small Intestine meridian.

Contra-Indications: None.

Houxi (Small Intestine 3) –
'Back Stream' – 後谿

This point is situated on the ulnar edge of the hand. This is the edge on the side of the little finger. It is in a depression next to the head of the fifth metacarpal bone at the base of the little finger.

Therapeutic Functions: This point helps to drain blockages from the section of the Small Intestine meridian running along the neck and shoulder so activating it can relieve pain in these areas. It also helps with the spiritual function of the Small Intestine so it is useful for those who have difficulty understanding concepts of right and wrong.

Qi Sensation: When activated you will feel a pressure in the location of the point. It is likely that you will also feel a pressure in the length of the Small Intestine meridian, particularly along the pathway which runs across the shoulders.

Contra-Indications: None.

Wangu (Small Intestine 4) –
'Wrist Bone' – 腕骨

Wangu is situated, as its name suggests, on the wrist in a depression between the bones. It is on the outside edge of the wrist in a depression between the fifth metacarpal and the triquetral bone. Note that many people locate this point poorly; take care to make sure you put this point in the correct place or you will be hitting Small Intestine 5 instead.

Therapeutic Functions: This is the Yuan source point of the Small Intestine meridian. It can be accessed and used to regulate all disorders of the Small Intestine. Its activation will also treat any disorders present along the length of the Small Intestine meridian pathway.

Qi Sensation: When activated you will feel a warm pressure that spreads out along the length of the meridian and sometimes over the whole hand.

Contra-Indications: None.

Jianzhen (Small Intestine 9) –
'True Shoulder' – 肩貞

Jianzhen is situated on the posterior aspect of the shoulder. It is not too difficult to locate though and it is a useful point so it is worth learning its location and uses. It is on the back of the shoulder, one thumb's breadth above the rear armpit fold when the arm is hanging down. If you use the opposite hand you may reach across your chest and feel for the point. It is tender when pressed.

Therapeutic Functions: This point is useful in any shoulder injuries. It is also a useful point for expelling environmental energies which may have invaded the Taiyang aspect of the meridian system. In the case of shoulder injury, you only need use this point on the affected side of the body.

Qi Sensation: When activated this point will radiate a tingling sensation over the shoulder and down the length of the arm towards the hand.

Contra-Indications: None.

Tianchuang (Small Intestine 16) – 'Window to Heaven' – 天窗

Tianchuang is on the outside edge of the sternocleidomastoid muscle. It is halfway up the neck, level with the larynx.

Therapeutic Functions: Tianchuang is named after its categorisation as a Heavenly Window point. These points are closely related to the consciousness body and in particular its connection to the realms of Heaven and Dao. It is the strongest point of the Small Intestine meridian for treating the spiritual aspect of the Small Intestine. It is also particularly useful for those who feel that they lack any kind of divine inspiration in life.

Qi Sensation: This point is particularly strange to experience when you first access it with your Yi. It will begin to tingle and then feel as if there is something exiting the neck at this point. With time it will feel as though there is steam leaving the point which floats up towards the sky.

Contra-Indications: None.

Tinggong (Small Intestine 19) – 'Place of Hearing' – 聽宮

Locate this point with your mouth open. It is situated in the depression next to the mid-point of the tragus by the ear.

Therapeutic Functions: This point is selected for those who have problems with their hearing. It can also be accessed and used by those who have difficulty listening; not just due to a physical issue but also through lack of interest or patience.

Qi Sensation: The warmth that radiates from this point when accessed radiates through into the ear and into the head.

Contra-Indications: None.

Useful Points on the Pericardium Meridian

Useful points along the pathway of the Pericardium meridian include: Tianchi (PC1), Quze (PC3), Neiguan (PC6), Daling (PC7), Laogong (PC8) and Zhongchong (PC9). These points are shown on the diagram of the Pericardium meridian in Figure 11.3.

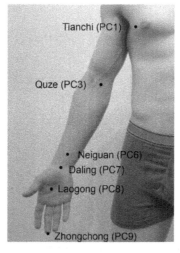

Figure 11.3: Pericardium Meridian Points

Tianchi (Pericardium 1) – 'Heavens Pool' – 天池

Tianchi is situated one thumb's breadth lateral to the nipple on men. It is not recommended as a point to use on women.

Therapeutic Functions: This is a Heavenly Window point meaning that it connects in to the consciousness aspect of a person. It can be accessed to help clear very deep traumas which have been buried deep within a person's consciousness. Due to its connection to the middle Dan Tien, this point can have profound effects on those who have deeply buried their emotions in the past. It is not recommended for use by women as disturbing the energy here can have a knock on effect to the health of the breasts.

Qi Sensation: Usually you will notice a feeling of warmth in the chest followed by an emotional release. This is nothing to worry about, just let it happen and within a few minutes you will feel okay again. The emotional release is just the body's way of reacting to a pent up information blockage which needs to get out of the energy system.

Contra-Indications: Not for use by women.

Quze (Pericardium 3) – 'Elbow Marsh' – 曲澤

This point is easily located on the elbow crease when the arm is slightly bent. It sits in the depression to the inside of the biceps tendon.

Therapeutic Functions: This point can help the Pericardium's function of clearing Heat from both the Heart and the Pericardium. It is also known to have strong calming effects upon those that are generally agitated as well as those who are emotionally uncomfortable in large groups of people.

Qi Sensation: Activation of this point will result in a feeling of warmth in the elbow. Those who were previously agitated should find that their mind becomes calm.

Contra-Indications: None.

Neiguan (Pericardium 6) – 'Internal Pass' – 內關

This point sits two thumbs' width from the inner wrist crease between the two prominent tendons.

Therapeutic Functions: This point is particularly useful for those with a tendency to feel nauseous; it can even be used when travelling for those who suffer with travel sickness. It is also known to reach the inner depths of a person's Heart after they have suffered the loss of a romantic partner. It can help ease somebody through the 'break-up' period.

It is also a very strong point used in the support of the energy of the Heart.

Qi Sensation: When activated this point will radiate with warmth. Curiously it is often accompanied by a feeling of warmth in the centre of the chest too, as the emotional centre begins to open up.

Contra-Indications: None.

Daling (Pericardium 7) – 'Large Mound' – 大陵

This point is the Yuan source point that you are likely already familiar with. It sits in the centre of the inner wrist crease between the two prominent tendons.

Therapeutic Functions: This point has similar functions to Shenmen (HE7) but with less strength. For those who are particularly sensitive to energy work you may wish to use this point before Shenmen (HE7). If it is not strong enough then select Shenmen (HE7).

Qi Sensation: When this point is observed, as in your earlier practices, it enabled you to make contact with the length of the meridian but now you are adding the power of your Qi via the breathing method outlined in the previous chapter. This will cause the point to fully activate which results in a comforting warmth which spreads out across the length of the meridian. You will usually also notice that your mind becomes very still when this point is activated as the emptiness at the centre of your Heart is directly contacted.

Contra-Indications: Not for use by people who suffer with depression of any sort.

Laogong (Pericardium 8) – 'Palace of Work' – 勞宮

Laogong sits in the centre of your hand. It is at the point where the ring finger makes contact with your palm when you make a fist.

Therapeutic Functions: This is the most important point for expelling Heat and pathogens of any sort from the upper body. It has a dredging effect upon all of the meridians of the arms as it has a direct connection with the branch of the thrusting meridian which travels deep through the inside of the arm. Remember this point. When using Laogong, it is wise to adjust your position so that your palms are facing away from you; turn the hands over as if you are pushing something in front of you.

Qi Sensation: Activating this point will result in a warm feeling that spreads out across the centre of the palm. After some time this point will begin to feel more solid and expansive; you will find that it is one of the largest meridian points on the body. It often feels as though it is swirling like some large whirlpool. This is a particularly strong point to make contact with.

Contra-Indications: Do not use this point if you feel cold in your body and limbs. It will take out Heat from the body so may run the risk of making excessively cold people colder.

Zhongchong (Pericardium 9) – *'Central Surging' –* 中衝

Zhongchong sits right at the very tip of the middle finger. This is the longest finger on your hand which acts much like a kind of organic 'exhaust pipe'.

Therapeutic Functions: This is the key point for dredging the Pericardium meridian to clear it of any imbalances and blockages that you have discovered. It is not as strong as Laogong (PC8) but does not drain the body of Heat so is more suitable for those who tend to have a low body temperature.

Qi Sensation: When this point is activated it can feel as though there is a gentle, warm breeze exiting the end of the finger. With time it will increase until it feels as though there is some invisible force tugging at the end of your finger. You may also feel pathogens travelling through the Pericardium meridian as they exit the body.

Contra-Indications: None.

Useful Points on the Triple Heater Meridian

Useful points along the pathway of the Triple Heater meridian include: Guanchong (TH1), Yangchi (TH4) and Waiguan (TH5). These points are shown on the diagram of the Triple Heater meridian in Figure 11.4.

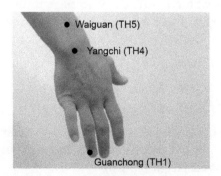

Figure 11.4: Triple Heater Meridian Points

Guanchong (Triple Heater 1) –
'Rushing Pass' – 關衝

Guanchong sits on the outer edge of the ring finger nail. It is situated level with the base of the nail and the outer edge.

Therapeutic Functions: This is the point activated to dredge any pathogen from the length of the Triple Heater meridian. It can be used despite the fact that the Triple Heater Qi actually flows the other way up the meridian. Opening this point is like taking the lid off a bottle so that the contents may escape.

Qi Sensation: When this point is activated you will feel energy leaving the end of the ring finger. It is as if there is steam rising from the point.

Contra-Indications: None.

Yangchi (Triple Heater 4) – 'Yang Pond' – 陽池

This point sits on the back of the wrist in the depression between the extensor tendons which run to the little and ring fingers. It is tricky to locate at first but easy to feel once you have found it as the point is tender when pressed.

Therapeutic Functions: This is the Yuan source point of the Triple Heater and so can be used to treat any imbalances within the Triple Heater. It is also something of a general treatment point as all of the other organs and elements of the energy body sit within one of the three energetic chambers of the Triple Heater. It is a personal favourite point of mine when treating those who suffer with low energy.

Qi Sensation: When activated this point will radiate warmth through the meridian. Those who are particularly sensitive to the movement of Qi within their body will also find that a warmth spreads throughout the whole body.

Contra-Indications: None.

Waiguan (Triple Heater 5) – 'Outer Pass' – 外關

Waiguan sits on the outer side of the forearm, two thumbs' distance from the wrist crease. It is in a depression between the radius and ulna bones. It is directly opposite Neiguan (PC6).

Therapeutic Functions: This point helps to pull any excess Heat from the body, from any organ or area of the meridian system. It also has a profound effect upon those suffering with any kind of sickness or fever. It can be used with Neiguan (PC6) to treat vomiting and nausea.

Qi Sensation: Activating this point will result in a feeling of pressure which radiates out from the point. It is much like an invisible finger is pressing onto the point during your practice. If there are many toxins in the Triple Heater meridian then this point may radiate a dull ache along the arm when activated. If this happens then dredge the meridian before returning to activate this point.

Contra-Indications: If the Triple Heater meridian is blocked then clear it before using this point.

Useful Points on the Spleen Meridian

Useful points along the pathway of the Spleen meridian include: Yinbai (SP1), Taibai (SP3), Gongsun (SP4), Sanyinjiao (SP6), Lougu (SP7), Diji (SP8), Yinlingquan (SP9), Xuehai (SP10) and Dabao (SP21). These points are shown on the diagram of the Spleen meridian in Figure 11.5.

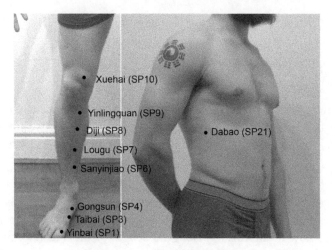

Figure 11.5: Spleen Meridian Points

Yinbai (Spleen 1) – 'Hiding White' – 隱白

Yinbai sits on the inside of the big toe nail. If you draw a line from the base of the nail and along the inner border, Yinbai sits where these two lines would meet.

Therapeutic Functions: This point can be used to dredge any imbalances or blockages from the length of the Spleen meridian.

Qi Sensation: When activated, Yinbai feels as though there is energy moving out of it. It is much like there is steam rising from the point.

Contra-Indications: None.

Taibai (Spleen 3) – 'Greater White' – 太白

Taibai is the Yun source point of the Spleen meridian. It sits on the inside edge of the foot in the depression just before the head of the first metatarsal bone.

Therapeutic Functions: This point strengthens the Spleen meaning that it treats any Spleen imbalance. Since many people have issues around the energy of their Spleen, this point is used a great deal. It also helps to strengthen the Pancreas which means it can be useful for those suffering with diabetes. It can also help to clear any Damp from the body due to the Spleen's close relationship to the Damp pathogen.

Qi Sensation: Activating this point causes a feeling of tingling to run all along the inside edge of the foot.

Contra-Indications: None.

Gongsun (Spleen 4) – 'Ancestor and Descendant' – 公孫

Gongsun sits on the inside edge of the foot in a depression next to the base of the first metatarsal bone. This point is very important within Daoist medical thought so ensure that you become familiar with its location.

Therapeutic Functions: The name of Gongsun links it to the line of ancestors which run right back to the legendary Yellow Emperor (Huangdi). It is the key point which connects the exterior of the body into the deep energies of the thrusting meridian. This point helps to create a strong upwards flow of information along the length of the thrusting meridian into the upper Dan Tien. It works in conjunction with Yongquan (KI1) to draw in the Qi of the planet which is then taken up into the body.

It can be used to treat any imbalances of the Spleen as well as any form of tiredness. Those who have a collapsed body posture will also benefit from this point as the surge of energy along the thrusting meridian will push the body upright.

Qi Sensation: This is one of the more difficult points to make contact with but with time and persistence it can be activated. It will result in a clear feeling of Qi running up the inside of the leg and then through the centre of the body. It is common for students to physically thrust their chests upwards towards the ceiling when this point is activated.

Contra-Indications: Do not use when pregnant.

Sanyinjiao (Spleen 6) – 'Meeting of the Three Yin' – 三陰交

Sanyinjiao is situated four fingers above the medial malleolus (the prominent bone on the inner ankle) close to the rear border of the tibia bone.

Therapeutic Functions: The energy of the Spleen, Liver and Kidneys meets at this point. It can be used to treat any imbalances within any of these organs; this makes it a very versatile and useful point to work with. This is also a strong point for depression of any sort. It uplifts the spirit and strengthens the resolve.

Qi Sensation: Activation at this point results in a tingling sensation which runs along the rear border of the tibia bone.

Contra-Indications: Do not use when pregnant.

Lougu (Spleen 7) – 'Leaking Place' – 漏谷

Lougu is situated four fingers' distance directly above Sanyinjiao (SP6) on the rear border of the tibia. It is in a tender depression.

Therapeutic Functions: This point stimulates the function of the Spleen which is connected into the muscles. It can help with anybody who has difficulty building muscle mass or for those who cannot gain weight no matter how much they eat. The name of the point suggests that it is a place on the body where nutritive energy may 'leak' out. Also useful for those with loose bowels.

Qi Sensation: Activating this point causes a feeling of tingling to run along the inside of the leg; often it radiates up to the top of the inner thigh as well.

Contra-Indications: None.

Diji (Spleen 8) – 'The Earth Pivot' – 地機

Diji is situated four fingers' distance below Yinlingquan (SP9) on the rear border of the tibia bone.

Therapeutic Functions: This point helps to strengthen the Earth aspect of the body and its relationship to the energetic functioning of the Spleen. It is useful for those with general digestive issues. It also has one very interesting function; if activated it will bring about great change in the Earth element. It will affect the Tai Yin aspect of the meridian system meaning that what was moist may now become dry and vice versa. If previous efforts to treat the Spleen were unsuccessful then try this point and see if the new situation is easier to work with!

Qi Sensation: Activating this point has the potential to change how you feel throughout the whole of your body.

Contra-Indications: Do not use this point unless you want to make a big change to the overall nature of your energetic balance.

Yinlingquan (Spleen 9) – 'Yin Hill Spring' – 陰陵泉

Yinlingquan is located just below the inside of the knee in a tender depression. If you run your finger up the rear border until it drops into a depression below the knee you will have located Yinlingquan.

Therapeutic Functions: This point is commonly used to treat any Spleen imbalance and to take Damp from the body. It is a strong point. It also has strong effect upon the part of your nature linked to empathy. It also has a strong effect upon the spiritual aspect of the Spleen meaning that it is good for those who worry too much.

Qi Sensation: This point will feel warm and as if there is pressure being exerted onto the inside of the knee when it is activated.

Contra-Indications: None.

Xuehai (Spleen 10) – 'Ocean of Blood' – 血海

Xuehai is located two thumbs' distance above the inner, top corner of the patella. It is sat in a tender depression.

Therapeutic Functions: This point has a strong connection to the health of the Blood and so any Blood related disorders can be treated with this point. These may include conditions such as anaemia through to irregular periods.

Qi Sensation: This point will feel very warm when activated. This warmth will radiate along the meridian around the area of the knee.

Contra-Indications: None.

Dabao (Spleen 21) – 'Great Enwrapping' – 大包

Dabao sits eight fingers' distance below the armpit on the mid-axillary line. It is in the space between the seventh and eighth rib.

Therapeutic Functions: This point regulates the Qi and Blood of the chest. Any weakness in energy around the chest, Heart and Lungs can be helped by accessing this point. It can also be used by those who find that they are emotionally incapable of relating to others – for those who feel 'emotionally repressed'.

Qi Sensation: Activating this point spreads a feeling of warmth throughout the whole of the chest cavity.

Contra-Indications: None.

Useful Points on the Stomach Meridian

Useful points along the pathway of the Stomach meridian include: Tianshu (ST25), Dubi (ST35), Zusanli (ST36), Fenglong (ST40), Jiexi (ST41), Chongyang (ST42) and Lidui (ST45). These points are shown on the diagram of the Stomach meridian in Figure 11.6.

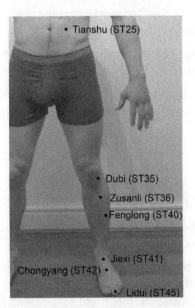

Figure 11.6: Stomach Meridian Points

Tianshu (Stomach 25) – 'The Heaven Pivot' – 天樞

This point sits two thumbs' distance lateral to the umbilicus.

Therapeutic Functions: This point regulates any imbalances of the Spleen, Stomach or digestive system in general. It is arguably the strongest point we can use in these practices for these types of imbalance. This point is also the pivot of the energy of Heaven, the consciousness. It can be of help to those who find that their moods are very quick to swing from one extreme to another; it literally brings us back to our 'centre' which is easy to remember as this point sits as the physical centre of the body.

Qi Sensation: Activating this point should cause the lower abdomen to warm up. Interestingly it is also common to feel a short line connecting the Tianshu point through the umbilicus; a line of the meridian system that is not mapped out on charts.

Contra-Indications: Do not use during pregnancy.

Dubi (Stomach 35) – 'Calf's Nose' – 犢鼻

This point is in the hollow depression near the outer, lower corner of the patella. This is a very easy point to locate.

Therapeutic Functions: This point is broadly indicated for any knee injuries or general blockages anywhere in the lower limbs.

Qi Sensation: This point should warm up very quickly upon activation and cause the entire knee to begin tingling as the Qi permeates the joint.

Contra-Indications: None.

Zusanli (Stomach 36) – 'Leg Three Miles' – 足三里

Zusanli sits four fingers' distance below Dubi (ST35) and one finger's distance from the outer border of the tibia bone.

Therapeutic Functions: This is the point you will likely have used already to practise meridian point activation. It has a strong effect upon the Yang Ming aspect of the meridian system and so strengthens the Qi and Blood. This point can be used whenever you like to generally strengthen the energy body.

Qi Sensation: Activating this point will cause tingling and heat to move from the point along the line of the meridian. If you practise for a while you will begin to feel these sensations move out into the whole body.

Contra-Indications: None.

Fenglong (Stomach 40) – 'Abundant Prosperity' – 豐隆

Fenglong is sat on the lower leg halfway between the lower border of the patella and ankle. It is halfway down the shin. It is also two fingers' distance from the outer border of the tibia bone.

Therapeutic Functions: This is a key point to access if there is Damp or Phlegm present anywhere in the body. Strangely it is also useful in the treatment of bad dreams.

Qi Sensation: Activating this point will cause tingling and heat to move from the point along the line of the meridian.

Contra-Indications: None.

Jiexi (Stomach 41) – 'Divided Stream' – 解谿

Jiexi sits in the centre of the anterior aspect of the ankle. It is in a clear depression between the two prominent tendons.

Therapeutic Functions: This point is useful for any ankle injuries. It can also be used for people suffering with depression of any kind. It helps to draw down Heat from the head.

Qi Sensation: Activating this point will cause tingling and heat to move from the point along the line of the meridian.

Contra-Indications: None.

Chongyang (Stomach 42) – 'Surging Yang' – 沖陽

Chongyang is two fingers' distance from Jiexi (ST41) on the top of the foot on its centreline. It is in a clear depression.

Therapeutic Functions: This is the Yuan source point of the Stomach meridian and so can be used to treat any imbalances of the Stomach. It is also useful in those with a low appetite.

Qi Sensation: Activating this point will cause tingling and heat to move from the point along the line of the meridian.

Contra-Indications: None.

Lidui (Stomach 45) –
'Powerful Exchange' – 厲兌

Lidui sits on the outer corner of the second toe nail. It is on the connecting point of the lines running from the base of the nail and the outer edge of the nail.

Therapeutic Functions: This is the key point to use when dredging the Stomach meridian of any blockages and imbalances you may have found. The Stomach meridian is prone to blockages so this is a useful point to become familiar with.

Qi Sensation: When this point is activated you will feel energy moving like steam out of the second toe. You may also be able to feel the blockages moving along the pathway of the Stomach meridian towards the foot as they attempt to exit the body.

Contra-Indications: None.

Useful Points on the Lung Meridian

Useful points along the pathway of the Lung meridian include: Yunmen (LU2), Chize (LU5), Lieque (LU7), Taiyuan (LU9) and Shaoshang (LU11). These points are shown on the diagram of the Lung meridian shown in Figure 11.7.

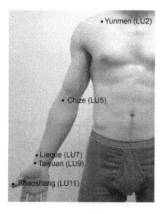

Figure 11.7: Lung Meridian Points

Yunmen (Lung 2) – 'Cloud Gate' – 雲門

Yunmen sits six fingers' breadth from the anterior midline. It is directly below the clavicle in a clear depression on the chest.

Therapeutic Functions: Yunmen is situated on the torso making it a little more difficult to connect with than many of the other points. I have included it in this list though due to its powerful function in clearing the mind. Yunmen has a strong connection to the energy of the Po. It can be used by those who feel that they are not clearly connected to the physical world; as if they are seeing everything through a thick mist. It also causes the energy of the Lungs to sink which has a soothing effect upon most Lung imbalances.

Qi Sensation: When Yunmen is activated it results in a tingling sensation around the point as well as the sensation that something is moving in the chest cavity. It is often described as feeling like mist floating around inside the Lungs and is quite likely the reason that this point got its name.

Contra-Indications: None.

Chize (Lung 5) – 'Outside Marsh' – 尺澤

Chize sits within the inner fold of the elbow crease on the outside of the biceps tendons. It is in a clear depression when the arm is slightly bent.

Therapeutic Functions: This point is categorised as the Water elemental point of the Lung meridian. It can help the Lungs if they are either 'too moist' or 'too dry' by regulating the fluids to which the Lungs relate. It is a useful point for any imbalance of the Lungs.

Qi Sensation: Activating Chize results in a slight feeling of pressure which radiates from the point down the length of the Lung meridian, usually only in the direction of the hand.

Contra-Indications: None.

Lieque (Lung 7) – 'Broken Sequence' – 列缺

Lieque can be tricky to locate so it is worth taking some time over this point. The point its two fingers' distance from the wrist crease between the brachioradialis and abductor pollicus longus tendons. It sits in a small groove. I have tried to avoid using technical anatomical terminology when describing the point locations but Lieque is difficult to locate without using the tendons in this area. I suggest you look up the tendons to help with the point's location.

Therapeutic Functions: This point can be used in the early stages of any environmental Qi invasion into the meridian system. It will help clear the pathogen before it enters deeper into the body. It can also be used in any imbalances within the Lung which are producing physical phlegm due to its function of relating to invading pathogens. Emotionally it has the interesting function of assisting those who are unable to grieve for a lost loved one. Activating this point can connect the consciousness to the memory of the event and enable it to manifest externally. Grieving is a healthy part of any loss; repressing it can lead to sickness.

Qi Sensation: Activating Lieque will send a feeling of pressure from the point along the pathway of the Lung meridian which runs through the forearm.

Contra-Indications: None.

Taiyuan (Lung 9) – 'The Great Abyss' – 太淵

Taiyuan is sat on the thumb side of the inner wrist crease. It is situated between the artery which you would use to read the pulse and the large tendon beside it (abductor pollicus longus).

Therapeutic Functions: Taiyuan is the Yuan source point of the Lung meridian. You should already have contacted this point to enable yourself to feel the length of the Lung meridian. Now that you are stimulating the point to activate it you will be able to use it to strengthen the Lungs. Strengthening the Lungs will help them to regain balance from any Lung condition. It can also be used to assist the body in clearing Phlegm which is present anywhere within the body.

Qi Sensation: Activating Taiyuan will first cause the length of the Lung meridian to appear as in your earlier practice. From here you will begin to feel a sense of pressure moving along the meridian. The Metal energy within the Lung meridian usually feels slightly contracting when Taiyuan is activated.

Contra-Indications: None.

Shaoshang (Lung 11) – 'Smaller Shang' – 少商

This point sits on the outside of the base of the thumb nail. It is on the point of intersection if two lines were drawn along the outer edge of the nail and the nail base.

Therapeutic Functions: Shaoshang is the key point used to expel any blockages or imbalances discovered along the length of the Lung meridian. It can also help to open up the Lungs for those who feel that their breathing is constricted.

Qi Sensation: Activating Shaoshang will feel as though there is an energy moving out of the point and escaping the thumb. It often feels as though there is smoke leaving the body as the pathogens begin to clear.

Contra-Indications: None.

Useful Points on the Large Intestine Meridian

Useful points along the pathway of the Large Intestine meridian include: Shangyang (LI1), Hegu (LI4), Yangxi (LI5), Shousanli (LI10), Quchi (LI11), Jianyu (LI15) and Yingxiang (LI20). These points are shown on the diagram of the Large Intestine meridian shown in Figure 11.8.

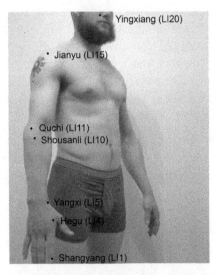

Figure 11.8: Large Intestine Meridian Points

Shangyang (Large Intestine 1) – 'Metal Yang' – 商陽

Shangyang sits on the outside of the index finger nail; the bottom nail corner nearest to the thumb. It is on the point of intersection if two lines were drawn along the outer edge of the nail and the nail base.

Therapeutic Functions: This is the point activated to clear blockages or imbalances which have been found along the length of the Large Intestine meridian. It is also useful for those who tend to hold grudges of any kind; within Daoist thought this is a sign of the emotional aspect of the Large Intestine being out of balance.

Qi Sensation: Activating Shangyang will feel as though there is an energy moving out of the point and escaping the index finger. It often feels as though there is smoke leaving the body as the pathogens begin to clear.

Contra-Indications: None.

Hegu (Large Intestine 4) – 'Connecting Valley' – 合谷

When the index finger and thumb are squeezed closed, Hegu sits at the highest point of the muscle which bulges between them.

Therapeutic Functions: Hegu is often known as the PPP, the Pain and Poo Point. Connecting with this point can help to alleviate pains due to stagnation anywhere on the body and can help to regulate either constipation or diarrhoea. Note that the pain alleviation to be had from this point is only temporary as it does not get to the root cause of the imbalance. This means that Hegu should be combined with other points in a single practice session. This is also an excellent point for anybody suffering with any kind of depression.

Qi Sensation: Be warned, activating Hegu can result in very swift bowel movements for those who have been blocked for a while!

Contra-Indications: This point should never be used during pregnancy.

Yangxi (Large Intestine 5) – 'Yang Stream' – 陽谿

With the thumb extended, this points sits in the large depression formed between the two tendons at the base of the thumb.

Therapeutic Functions: This point can be used for any sensations of Heat in the guts as well as constipation. It is also useful for those wishing to move stagnant food which is sitting within the colon; signs of this include bad breath, strong smelling sweat and body odour as well as excessive flatulence.

Qi Sensation: Activating Yangxi results in a feeling of warmth in the area of the point which spreads out to cover the whole wrist area.

Contra-Indications: None.

Shousanli (Large Intestine 10) – 'Arm Three Miles' – 手三里

This point is two thumbs' width from Quchi (LI11). It is on the line connecting Quchi (LI11) to Yangxi (LI5). The point sits in a clear depression.

Therapeutic Functions: Shousanli activates the abundant Qi aspect of the Yang Ming aspect of the meridian system. For this reason it is an effective Qi tonic along with Zusanli (ST36). This point affects the whole Yang Ming aspect and so is also helpful in treating Stomach disorders.

Qi Sensation: Activating this point will result in a feeling of warmth which spreads out form the elbow along the line of the Large Intestine meridian.

Contra-Indications: None.

Quchi (Large Intestine 11) – 'Elbow Pond' – 曲池

When the arm is bent, Quchi sits on the outer end of the elbow crease.

Therapeutic Functions: Quchi is a strong Heat removing point due to its Yang Ming aspect of alleviating excesses within both the Qi and Blood. This point was also one of the traditional Ghost points and so is indicated in cases of spiritual possession!

Qi Sensation: Activation of Quchi results in a feeling of warmth flowing out from the point along the length of the Large Intestine meridian.

Contra-Indications: This point should not be used on people who are lacking in energy or for those who have difficulty warming their body.

Jianyu (Large Intestine 15) – 'Shoulder Bone' – 肩髃

This point is most easily located with the arm lifted. Jianyu sits in the clear depression in front of the acromion (the lump on the outside of your shoulder).

Therapeutic Functions: This point is used extensively in any kind of shoulder injury or pain. It removes environmental pathogens from the upper body and so is useful in arm pain which is worsened when out in Cold, Damp or Windy environments. It is often listed as a strong point for draining excess Heat from the hands and feet.

Qi Sensation: Activation of Jianyu will cause the area to warm up. With time this warmth will begin to spread out to cover the entire shoulder and upper back.

Contra-Indications: None.

Yingxiang (Large Intestine 20) – 'Welcome Fragrance' – 迎香

This point sits on the outside corner of the nose, near the nostrils.

Therapeutic Functions: This point has a strong effect upon the nose, our sense of smell and the sinuses.

Qi Sensation: It is common to feel this point when working with any of the Large Intestine points; when focused upon it tingles. With time it turns into a sense of itchiness which you always resist the urge to scratch.

Contra-Indications: None.

Useful Points on the Kidney Meridian

Useful points on the Kidney meridian include: Yongquan (KI1), Taixi (KI3), Zhaohai (KI6) and Fuliu (KI7). These points are shown on the diagram of the Kidney meridian shown in Figure 11.9 (see below for an explanation as to why the numbering may seem odd).

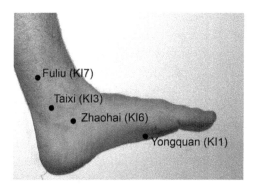

Figure 11.9: Kidney Meridian Points

Yongquan (Kidney 1) –
'Bubbling Spring' – 涌泉

This point sits on the sole of the foot. It is roughly a third of the way between the base of the second toe and the heel. It is pretty central to the foot. It can easily be found upon palpation as the point should feel tender with pressure, as if you are pushing on a bruise.

Therapeutic Functions: The Kidney meridian does not tend to fill with blockages and imbalances as the other meridians do; instead it tends to be deficient. This being said, if there are blockages here then this point can be used to expel them. It is more commonly used to draw in excess energy from the Earth and to pull energy away from the head. If it feels as if there is too much pressure in your skull then this point is useful. This point is also useful for those with high blood pressure.

Qi Sensation: As the name of this point suggests, activating it causes a feeling of bubbles under the base of the foot. It is much like standing over one of the air holes in the bottom of a Jacuzzi. With time this feeling moves up along the length of the Kidney meridian although it usually becomes less distinct at the height of the knee.

Contra-Indications: This point should never be used during pregnancy.

Taixi (Kidney 3) – 'Maximum Stream' – 太谿

This point sits in a clear depression between the inner malleolus and the Achilles tendon. This is one of the easiest points to locate.

Therapeutic Functions: This is the Yuan source point of the Kidney meridian. It is the strongest point on the Kidney meridian for treating Kidney Yin deficiency although it can also be used to treat any Kidney imbalances. It is a useful point for any lower back weaknesses due to the internal pathway of the Kidney meridian.

Qi Sensation: Activating this point should bring a feeling of warmth that moves up along the pathway of the Kidney meridian as well as warmth in the lower back due to the connection between the Kidneys and the Ming Fire. It is common for this point to feel as though it is pulsing after it has been activated for some time.

Contra-Indications: None.

Zhaohai (Kidney 6) – 'Shining Sea' – 照海

The numbering of the points on the Kidney meridian can appear quite strange at first but this is due to a small loop that the meridian makes on the ankle. Zhaohai is situated in the depression immediately below the inner malleolus.

Therapeutic Functions: This is another point on the Kidney meridian used to nourish the Yin aspect of the Kidneys. It is also useful for those with an excess of pathogenic Dryness within the body.

Qi Sensation: Activating this point will cause a feeling of warmth to radiate from the point out along the Kidney meridian.

Contra-Indications: None.

Fuliu (Kidney 7) – 'Repeating Current' – 復溜

Fuliu sits two thumbs' distance above Taixi (KI3). It is next to the Achilles tendon.

Therapeutic Functions: This is the key point upon the Kidney meridian used to treat Kidney Yang deficient imbalances.

Qi Sensation: Activating this point will cause a feeling of warmth to radiate from the point out along the Kidney meridian.

Contra-Indications: None.

Useful Points on the Bladder Meridian

Useful points on the Bladder meridian include: Zanzhu (BL2), Kunlun (BL60), Shenmai (BL62) and Jingu (BL64). These points are shown on the diagram of the Bladder meridian shown in Figure 11.10.

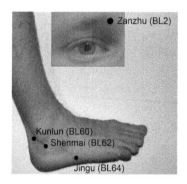

Figure 11.10: Bladder Meridian Points

Zanzhu (Bladder 2) – 'Collected Bamboo' – 攢竹

Zanzhu sits in a small depression upon the inner edge of the eyebrow.

Therapeutic Functions: A useful point for expelling the Wind pathogen from the head and for general imbalance within the energy of the eyes.

Qi Sensation: Activating this point will result in a feeling of tingling in the eyebrow which will begin to spread to the back of the eyes.

Contra-Indications: None.

Kunlun (Bladder 60) – 'Kunlun Mountains' – 昆侖

Kunlun sits behind the ankle joint in a clear depression between the outer malleolus and the Achilles tendon. It is opposite Taixi (KI3) which sits on the inside of the ankle.

Therapeutic Functions: This point is useful to clear any painful blockages or imbalances which may sit along the pathway of the Bladder meridian.

Qi Sensation: Activating this point will bring a feeling of warmth in the area of the point which will spread along the line of the Bladder meridian. It is also common to have dull aches appear along the section of the Bladder meridian which runs alongside the spine if there are imbalances present here.

Contra-Indications: Not to be used in pregnancy.

Shenmai (Bladder 62) – 'Outstretched Meridian' – 申脈

Shenmai sits in a clear depression directly beneath the outer malleolus.

Therapeutic Functions: This is the key point on the Bladder meridian used to treat any imbalances in the energy of the Bladder. It is also highly effective at taking Wind out of the body, especially if it has invaded the Tai Yang aspect of the body.

Qi Sensation: Activating this point will result in a feeling of warmth which spreads out over the foot.

Contra-Indications: None.

Jingu (Bladder 64) – 'Capital Bone' – 京骨

Jingu sits on the outer edge of the foot in a depression directly in front of the clear boney prominence formed by the tuberosity of the fifth metatarsal bone.

Therapeutic Functions: This is the Yuan source point of the Bladder meridian. It can be used to treat any imbalances of the Bladder since it strengthens its energy. For some unknown reason it is also more effective at dredging the length of the Bladder meridian than the final Bladder point which sits on the little toe. Experience has shown me that pathogens from the Bladder meridian do not exit from the fingers and toes, as in the case of the other meridians (with the exception of the Kidney meridian). Instead we can use Jingu as our dredging point.

Qi Sensation: When Jingu is activated you should begin to feel energy exiting the point. It is much like steam leaving through the point. You may also become aware of the pathogens you are trying to clear moving along the line of the Bladder meridian.

Contra-Indications: None.

Useful Points on the Liver Meridian

Useful points on the Liver meridian include: Dadun (LV1), Xingjian (LV2) and Taichong (LV3). These points are shown on the diagram of the Liver meridian shown in Figure 11.11.

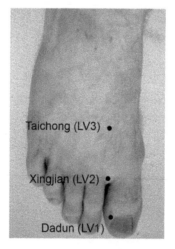

Figure 11.11: Liver Meridian Points

Dadun (Liver 1) – 'Big Mound' – 大敦

Dadun sits on the inner corner of the big toe nail.

Therapeutic Functions: Dadun is the most effective point for dredging the Liver meridian of any imbalances or blockages you may have found during your exploration of the meridian system.

Qi Sensation: Activating this point will result in a sensation much like steam leaving the end of the big toe. You will also likely become aware of pathogens moving along the length of the Liver meridian.

Contra-Indications: None.

Xingjian (Liver 2) – 'Moving Between' – 行間

This point sits on the top of the foot between the big toe and the second toe. It is half your little finger's distance from the web between these two toes.

Therapeutic Functions: This is the key point for taking Heat out of the liver so it is good for treating the conditions of Liver Fire and Liver Yang rising.

Qi Sensation: Activating this point will result in a feeling of coolness between the first and second toes.

Contra-Indications: Do not use this point if you have low energy levels or feel cold a lot of the time. It is quite a draining point and should only be used in conditions of excessive Heat.

Taichong (Liver 3) – 'Great Thrusting' – 太沖

Taichong sits on the top of the foot. If you slide your finger from Xingjian (LV2) up towards the ankle between the metatarsal bones you will feel a depression where the metatarsal bones meet. It is a very distinct depression which is easy to locate; this depression is the location of Taichong.

Therapeutic Functions: This is the Yuan source point of the Liver meridian and the key point used in the treatment of all Liver conditions as it has a general rebalancing effect upon the Liver. It also has a close relationship to the consciousness aspect of the Hun which is said to move through the pulse which can be felt at this point. Any irregularities in the Hun can be treated with this point.

Qi Sensation: Activating this point results in a feeling of warmth which spreads outwards along the line of the Liver meridian. It is also common to feel the pulse here as your awareness is drawn deeper into contact with the point.

Contra-Indications: None.

Useful Points on the Gall Bladder Meridian

Useful points on the Gall Bladder meridian include: Fengchi (GB20), Jianjing (GB21), Yanglingquan (GB34), Qinxu (GB40) and Zuqiaoyin (GB44). These points are shown on the diagram of the Gall Bladder meridian shown in Figure 11.12.

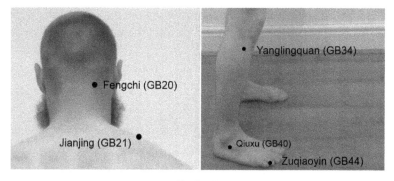

Figure 11.12: Gall Bladder Meridian Points

Fengchi (Gall Bladder 20) – 'Wind Pool' – 風池

Fengchi sits in the depression below the occiputs. To be honest, this point is quite large and so you do not have to be too exact when accessing this point with your Yi. Obviously this is not the case when using a needle in the case of acupuncturists though!

Therapeutic Functions: This point is the key point for expelling Wind from the body. It is also useful in any painful blockages around the head, neck and shoulders. Fengchi has a strong effect upon the Shao Yang aspect of the meridian system meaning that it can free up stagnation anywhere in the body; it is especially strong when treating stagnation along the side of the torso.

Qi Sensation: Activating this point will result in a feeling of coolness in the area under the occiputs. If there is excessive Wind to be expelled from the body then you may feel it exiting from this point. It is much like dredging the meridians, like steam escaping from the point.

Contra-Indications: None.

Jianjing (Gall Bladder 21) – 'Shoulder Well' – 肩井

This point sits midway between the seventh cervical vertebrae and the acromion. Jianjing sits at the highest point of the trapezius muscle.

Therapeutic Functions: This point is useful in treating shoulder injuries or pain of any kind. It also drops Qi down through the body making it useful for those who feel as though they have too much energetic pressure in the upper body or head. It can also help to free up the energy of the Lungs for those who feel that they cannot breathe very easily.

Qi Sensation: When this point is activated, any tension in the shoulders will show up as a dull ache. You will also likely be able to feel energy moving down through the chest into the abdomen.

Contra-Indications: Never use when pregnant. Do not use if you have organ prolapse of any kind or haemorrhoids.

Yanglingquan (Gall Bladder 34) – 'Yang Hill Spring' – 陽陵泉

This point is quite tricky to locate at first. For this reason I suggest you see the Gall Bladder meridian diagram in Figure 11.12 for assistance. It sits in a depression one thumb's distance in front of and below the head of the fibula. Make sure you correctly identify the fibula and do not use the tibia by accident which is a common error.

Therapeutic Functions: Yanglingquan is the most important point for treating any physical injury in the body. It causes any stagnation in the tendons to clear up due to the function of the Shao Yang aspect of the meridian system. Strangely it is also useful for those who are very shy despite the fact that this function would more logically apply to the Kidney and Bladder meridians.

Qi Sensation: When this point is activated you will feel a pressure which spreads out into the surrounding area. If you have any physical injuries you may also feel pressure or Qi movement in these areas.

Contra-Indications: None.

Qiuxu (Gall Bladder 40) – 'Ruined Hill' – 丘墟

Qiuxu is located diagonally down and forward from the outer malleolus. It is one finger's distance from the front lower corner of this bone in a clear depression.

Therapeutic Functions: This point is an important point on the Gall Bladder meridian. Activating this point helps to treat any general aches and pains which sit along the side of the body or head. It is also useful as an adjunct to other points if you wish to strengthen their function. For example: You may use a point on the Lung meridian to help strengthen the Lung Qi and then use Qiuxu to help strengthen this process. Some styles of Acupuncture use this point often for this reason. It is also indicated in many texts for assisting those who have difficulty making decisions.

Qi Sensation: When this point is activated you will feel general warmth in the area of the point which will spread along the line of the meridian.

Contra-Indications: None.

Zuqiaoyin (Gall Bladder 44) – *'Foot Yin Holes' –* 足竅陰

Zuqiaoyin sits at the outer corner of the base of the fourth toe nail.

Therapeutic Functions: This is the key point for clearing any imbalances or blockages from the length of the Gall Bladder meridian. The Yin Holes of the point's name refer to the eyes, nose, mouth and ears. Through the principle of Yin (below) balancing Yang (above) this point can be accessed to help sort out any imbalances within these sensory organs.

Qi Sensation: When Zuqiaoyin is activated you will feel energy moving out of this point and leaving the body like steam.

Contra-Indications: None.

Useful Points on the Governing Meridian

Useful points on the governing meridian include: Mingmen (GV4) and Baihui (GV20). These points are shown on the diagram of the governing meridian shown in Figure 11.13.

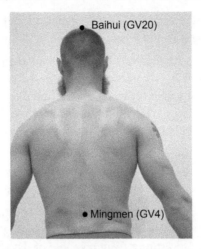

Figure 11.13: Governing Meridian Points

Mingmen (Governing Meridian 4) – 'Gate of Ming' – 命門

Mingmen sits on the midline of the lower back directly below the second lumbar vertebra. Mingmen is so useful that it is worth taking the time and effort to locate it. For the first few times it may be useful to get a friend to locate it for you and massage the point until you are able to find it easily with your awareness.

Therapeutic Functions: Mingmen has already been discussed in Chapter 7. This point can be accessed to treat any conditions of the Kidneys and Jing as well as general tiredness or hypo-function of any of the organs. It is especially useful for those with reproductive issues and for those who have difficulty keeping their body warm. Many people would benefit from activating this point.

Qi Sensation: Activating this point should warm up the lower back. With time this warmth should increase a great deal until the entire body is hot. It is common to be soaked in sweat after successfully activating this point.

Contra-Indications: None.

Baihui (Governing Meridian 20) – 'The Hundred Meetings' – 百會

Baihui sits directly on top of the head. If you wish to locate it accurately then fold the lobes of the ears over. The highest point of the folded ears can then be used as a marker. Slide your hands up to the top of your head from the top of the ears and where they meet is Baihui.

Therapeutic Functions: Baihui can be accessed to regulate the energy of the thrusting meridian. It balances the energy which runs through our core which makes it useful for many conditions. For the purposes of our practice we can use it to treat any imbalances of the Brain or Marrow as well as a general regulating point for the energies of the five elements.

Qi Sensation: Activating this point will result in the feeling of having a hole in the top of the head. With practice you can even feel it breathing energy in and out in time with your physical respiration.

Contra-Indications: Be respectful of this point. If you have any sensations of pressure building in the top of the head then stop immediately. Your focus is most likely too strong. Wait a couple of days and then try again with a more relaxed level of focus. Not for use by those with any kind of depression.

Useful Points on the Conception Meridian

Useful points on the conception meridian include: Huiyin (CO1), Guanyuan (CO4), Qihai (CO6), Shanzhong (CO17), Tiantu (CO22) and Chengjiang (CO24). These points are shown on the diagrams of the conception meridian shown in Figure 11.14.

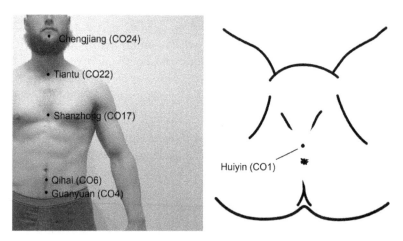

Figure 11.14: Conception Meridian Points

Huiyin (Conception Meridian 1) –
'Meeting of Yin' – 會陰

Huiyin sits in the centre of the perineum at the midway between the anus and the genitalia. It is tender when pressed. Due to its location, it is rarely used within therapies such as massage or acupuncture but is a useful for point for the practices in this book.

Therapeutic Functions: This is an important point on the meridian system since it is the origin of the 'small water wheel of Qi' within practices such as Nei Gong. It has a close relationship to both the lower Dan Tien and the storehouse of the essence. It can be accessed and used in practice when all other treatments have failed as it is much like a reset button on the body. It also said to be one of the exit points for the wandering Po meaning that it is useful in conditions of emotional shock and even insomnia. Due to its locality it is also useful in helping pain and disease of the genitalia and anus.

Qi Sensation: Activating this point causes warmth to spread across the area of the perineum, the genitalia and up through the lower part of the thrusting meridian. It is also likely to cause sexual arousal when activated due to the movement of essence which is being generated. It is important that you do not have sex for at least an hour after activating this point though as it will heavily drain the Jing.

Contra-Indications: Do not have sex for at least an hour after activating this point.

Guanyuan (Conception Meridian 4) –
'Gate of the Congenital' – 關元

Guanyuan sits on the anterior midline of the lower abdomen four fingers' distance from the lower border of the umbilicus (belly button).

Therapeutic Functions: This is an extremely important point in the treatment of the Kidneys, essence and any imbalances in the energy of the Uterus. Very useful for those who feel tired no matter how much they rest.

Qi Sensation: When Guanyuan is activated a warm wave will spread across the lower abdomen and into the area of the groin. It is also common to become sexually aroused after activating this point although having sex within an hour after accessing this point will result in a heavy drain of the Jing.

Contra-Indications: Do not have sex for at least an hour after activating this point.

Qihai (Conception Meridian 6) – 'Sea of Qi' – 氣海

Qihai sits two fingers' distance below the lower border of the umbilicus (belly button) on the anterior midline of the lower abdomen.

Therapeutic Functions: Qihai consolidates the Qi of the body when activated. It has a strengthening effect upon every organ of the body and so is a useful point to focus upon. Interestingly this point is also known within the Daoist tradition as the false Dan Tien. It is named this as many people focus here by accident when trying to make contact with the lower Dan Tien using their awareness. I teach a great deal of people on a regular basis, many of these people come from outside schools and other teachers of Qi Gong. I would estimate that around 80–90 per cent of them are focusing on Qihai when they think they are focusing upon the lower Dan Tien. While this may bring health benefits as this point is activated it does not bring any of the attainments in skill associated with effective lower Dan Tien work.

Qi Sensation: Activating this point will bring feelings of warmth and pressure in the lower abdomen. This is the sensation many Qi Gong practitioners mistakenly think is the awakening of the lower Dan Tien.

Contra-Indications: None.

Shanzhong (Conception Meridian 17) – 'Centre of the Chest' – 膻中

As the name of the point suggests, Shanzhong sits at the centre of the chest. It is level with the nipples on men. The point is a little difficult to locate on women; palpate to locate the top of the sternum. There are ridges along the sternum if you move your fingers downwards. Shanzhong sits within the fourth depression on the anterior midline.

Therapeutic Functions: This point is used to treat overly emotional people due to its strong connection to the Heart, Pericardium and middle Dan Tien. It is also useful in the treatment of any imbalances of the breasts. I have included it within this book as I have found it the most useful point to activate for those who find they are very tight in the chest and for those who have difficulty working with their breath in Daoist practices.

Tightness of the chest and poor breathing is usually seen as a reflection of emotional debris stuck in the centre of the chest or the middle Dan Tien region.

Qi Sensation: Activating this point brings a feeling of warmth in the chest and breasts. It is also common for those working with this point to experience strong emotional releases. Do not worry about this, it is quite natural, just allow it to happen and do not analyse the nature of the emotional release too much.

Contra-Indications: None.

Tiantu (Conception Meridian 22) – 'Tiantu' – 天突

Tiantu sits in the centre of the suprasternal fossa, the soft depression at the base of your throat above the boney prominence of the sternum.

Therapeutic Functions: Tiantu is used to expel any blockages in the throat you feel may be linked to emotional imbalances. Due to its categorisation as a Heavenly Window point, Tiantu can help to connect you to the power of Heaven. It is useful for those who feel that life is overly difficult and that they are prone to excessive bad luck.

Qi Sensation: Activating this point should free up the breathing. You should feel very relaxed and as if you can breathe more deeply than before.

Contra-Indications: If you have a build-up of pressure at this point during practice then stop. You are using too much focus. Wait a couple of days and then try again with a more gentle level of focus.

Chengjiang (Conception Meridian 24) – 'Fluid Container' – 承漿

Chengjiang sits in the centre of the mentolabial groove, the depression between your lower lip and your chin.

Therapeutic Functions: This point is classically used to treat any disorders of the face and neck. I was also taught that it was useful in the treatment of the speech. This may be the physical act of speech, making the point useful for those with a speech impediment, or for those who cannot speak the truth. Those who cannot help exaggerating or lying may use this point to change the spiritual root of their speech.

Qi Sensation: Activating this point brings a feeling of warmth which spreads across the chin. As the name of the point suggests, it is common for you to also begin producing a lot of saliva when this point is activated.

Contra-Indications: None.

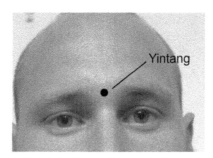

Figure 11.15: Yintang

Extra Points

Yintang – 'Hall of Impression' – 印堂

Yintang sits at the classical location of the 'third eye', between the eyebrows on the anterior midline of the face. It is not part of any of the meridians and is classified as one of the extra points of the body.

Therapeutic Functions: Yintang connects in to the upper Dan Tien and as such gives us a connection to the higher functions of our consciousness. It is used extensively in the mid-level stages of Daoist meditation but for the purposes of those following the practices outlined in this book it should be used to calm the mind.

Qi Sensation: If this point activates you should feel as if there is a hole between your eyebrows. You will also become aware of the energy body 'breathing' in and out through this point.

Contra-Indications: Do not use this point if you have any kind of tendency towards mental abnormalities or any kind of depression as it will make it worse. If pressure begins to build up at this point then stop, wait a couple of days and then try again. Your focus was too strong which led too much Qi to this point, use a more gentle focus so that the point is activated more gently.

The following two points exist within the external etheric body. To be able to connect with these two points requires having reached a very high standard of Nei Gong practice. They have been included here for those few practitioners who are able to reach this stage in their practice. These two points are known as the Heaven Linking Point and the Earth Linking Point. They are shown in Figure 11.16.

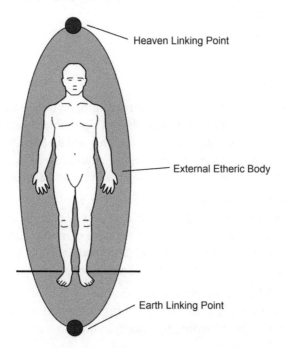

Figure 11.16: Heaven and Earth Linking Points

Heaven Linking Point

This point sits above the head. The distance can vary from person to person so it may take some exploration to locate. Only very advanced practitioners will be able to locate this point. Even fewer will be able to work with and activate this point. It is included here largely for completion purposes as those advanced enough to use this point should have a high degree of internal harmony already.

Therapeutic Functions: Contacting this point brings a stronger connection to the force of Yang which emanates down from Heaven. This is a point of divine inspiration, a point of direct connection to the force of Dao as it enters the realm of man and flows through us. It is a point commonly connected with through long-time practice of circle walking, one of the oldest Daoist internal practices which is rooted in shamanic traditions.

Qi Sensation: Activating this point is usually accompanied by a ball of white light which can be seen with both the mind and physical eyes. It shoots quickly from the Heaven Linking Point down through the body into the ground.

Contra-Indications: None.

Earth Linking Point

This point sits roughly 12 inches under the ground below our feet. Only very advanced practitioners will be able to locate this point. Even fewer will be able to work with and activate this point. It is included here largely for completion purposes as those advanced enough to use this point should have a high degree of internal harmony already.

Therapeutic Functions: This is the point whereby the lower Dan Tien connects energetically with the force of the planet. It is a point of nourishing connection with the great Yin force of mother Earth. It is used in the higher levels of arts such as Nei Gong and Taijiquan where the root is strengthened through connection of this point to the lower Dan Tien.

Qi Sensation: When this point activates the body will begin to tremble at a very high frequency. The Dan Tien will begin to rotate of its own accord and so you will feel a swirling movement in the lower abdomen.

Contra-Indications: None.

Hands and Feet

Figures 11.17 and 11.18 show close up views of points on the hands and feet that have already been discussed in this chapter. The figures have been included here to help in the location of these points.

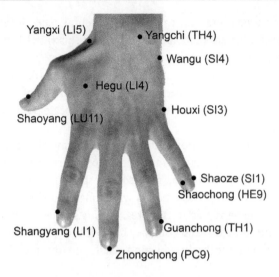

Figure 11.17: Points on the Hand

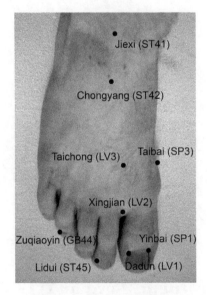

Figure 11.18: Points on the Foot

Treatment of Points on the Back

I have kept meridian points which sit on the back of the body apart from the rest of the meridian commentaries. This is primarily because many of their functions are the same: They work to nourish the energy of the body part or organ attached to the intervertebral space level with that particular point. Where there are exceptions to this rule I have indicated within the commentary for that particular point.

The points of the back I have selected for this book are taken from the Governing and Bladder meridians (for the positions of the points see Figure 11.19). A discussion of how to assess and locate points of the back is included in Chapter 9.

When activated, these points begin to feel warm. After some time the warmth felt here will spread along the line of the meridian upon which they sit. It is also common for a person to spontaneously jerk upright during the assessment of these points which may cause a cracking sound to come from the vertebrae in this area. This is similar to the sound you get when a chiropractor works on your back. It is nothing to worry about and simply shows the body adjusting itself into the most natural and healthy position.

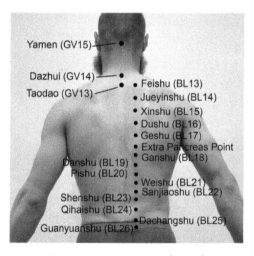

Figure 11.19: Points on the Back

Yamen (Governing Meridian 15) – 'Mute Gate' – 啞門

Yamen sits on the midline of the back of your neck between the first and second cervical vertebrae in the depression beneath the base of the skull.

Therapeutic Functions: Activating this point helps to work with the energy of the tongue. This can help those with speech impediments such as a stutter. It is also useful for those who find themselves always saying the wrong things. Those people who end up inadvertently hurting people's feelings may benefit from activation of this point.

Contra-Indications: None.

Dazhui (Governing Meridian 14) – 'Big Hammer' – 大椎

Dazhui sits on the midline of the back between the seventh cervical vertebrae and the first thoracic vertebrae. This places it at the base of your neck.

Therapeutic Functions: Activating this point helps to treat imbalances along the length of the spine. It is particularly useful for those with unhealthy posture caused by twists in the spine. It is also useful for those with general back pain not local to any one particular area.

Contra-Indications: None.

Taodao (Governing Meridian 13) – 'The Way to Happiness' – 陶道

Taodao sits on the rear midline between the first and second thoracic vertebrae.

Therapeutic Functions: Activating Taodao enables the clearing function of the middle Dan Tien to awaken. It can be used by those who feel that they have emotional debris stuck in the area of their chest. This is a very clear sensation which many people describe after having a severe emotional shock.

Contra-Indications: None.

Feishu (Bladder Meridian 13) – 'Lung Delivery Point' – 肺俞

Feishu sits either side of the spine. It is two fingers' distance from the spine between the third and fourth thoracic vertebrae.

Therapeutic Functions: Activating this point sends more Qi to the Lungs strengthening their energetic and physical functions.

Contra-Indications: None.

Jueyinshu (Bladder Meridian 14) – 'Jueyin Division Delivery Point' – 厥陰俞

Jueyinshu sits either side of the spine. It is two fingers' distance from the spine between the fourth and fifth thoracic vertebrae.

Therapeutic Functions: Activating this point sends more Qi to the Pericardium strengthening its energetic and physical functions.

Contra-Indications: None.

Xinshu (Bladder Meridian 15) – 'Heart Delivery Point' – 心俞

Xinshu sits either side of the spine. It is two fingers' distance from the spine between the fifth and sixth thoracic vertebrae.

Therapeutic Functions: Activating this point sends more Qi to the Heart strengthening its energetic and physical functions.

Contra-Indications: None.

Dushu (Bladder Meridian 16) – 'Governing Delivery Point' – 督俞

Dushu sits either side of the spine. It is two fingers' distance from the spine between the sixth and seventh thoracic vertebrae.

Therapeutic Functions: Activating this point helps the governing meridian's function of sending Qi to the other meridians. It is useful for those who often feel very drained for no obvious reason. Often this tiredness is due to the Spleen or Kidneys but if treatment here fails then Dushu may be used.

Contra-Indications: None.

Geshu (Bladder Meridian 17) – 'Diaphragm Delivery Point' – 膈俞

Geshu sits either side of the spine. It is two fingers' distance from the spine between the seventh and eighth thoracic vertebrae.

Therapeutic Functions: Activating this point sends more Qi to the diaphragm strengthening its energetic and physical functions. It is useful for those who have tightness in the lower part of their chest although obviously this is often treated through the Lungs. Angry stagnant emotional information also sticks to the diaphragm so this point can help those trying to clear old feelings of anger and resentment.

Contra-Indications: None.

Extra Pancreas Point

This point sits two fingers' distance from the spine on either side between the eighth and ninth thoracic vertebrae. It is often omitted from Chinese medicine texts.

Therapeutic Functions: Activating this point sends more Qi to the Pancreas strengthening its physical function.

Contra-Indications: None.

Ganshu (Bladder Meridian 18) – 'Liver Delivery Point' – 肝俞

Ganshu sits either side of the spine. It is two fingers' distance from the spine between the ninth and tenth thoracic vertebrae.

Therapeutic Functions: Activating this point sends more Qi to the Liver strengthening its energetic and physical functions.

Contra-Indications: None.

Danshu (Bladder Meridian 19) – 'Gall Bladder Delivery Point' – 膽俞

Danshu sits either side of the spine. It is two fingers' distance from the spine between the tenth and eleventh thoracic vertebrae.

Therapeutic Functions: Activating this point sends more Qi to the Gall Bladder strengthening its energetic and physical functions.

Contra-Indications: None.

Pishu (Bladder Meridian 20) – 'Spleen Delivery Point' – 脾俞

Pishu sits either side of the spine. It is two fingers' distance from the spine between the eleventh and twelfth thoracic vertebrae.

Therapeutic Functions: Activating this point sends more Qi to the Spleen strengthening its energetic and physical functions.

Contra-Indications: None.

Weishu (Bladder Meridian 21) – 'Stomach Delivery Point' – 胃俞

Weishu sits either side of the spine. It is two fingers' distance from the spine between the twelfth thoracic vertebra and the first lumbar vertebra.

Therapeutic Functions: Activating this point sends more Qi to the Stomach strengthening its energetic and physical functions.

Contra-Indications: None.

Sanjiaoshu (Bladder Meridian 22) – 'Triple Heater Delivery Point'– 三焦俞

Ganshu sits either side of the spine. It is two fingers' distance from the spine between the first and second lumbar vertebrae.

Therapeutic Functions: Activating this point sends more Qi to the Triple Heater strengthening its energetic and physical functions.

Contra-Indications: None.

Shenshu (Bladder Meridian 23) – 'Kidney Delivery Point' – 腎俞

Shenshu sits either side of the spine. It is two fingers' distance from the spine between the second and third lumbar vertebrae.

Therapeutic Functions: Activating this point sends more Qi to the Kidneys strengthening their energetic and physical functions.

Contra-Indications: None.

Qihaishu (Bladder Meridian 24) – 'Sea of Energy Delivery Point' – 氣海俞

Qihaishu sits either side of the spine. It is two fingers' distance from the spine between the third and fourth lumbar vertebrae.

Therapeutic Functions: Activating this point sends more Qi to the lower Dan Tien strengthening its energetic function of converting Jing to Qi. This point is usually used only by those who study Daoist alchemical methods.

Contra-Indications: None.

Dachangshu (Bladder Meridian 25) – 'Large Intestine Delivery Point' – 大腸俞

Dachangshu sits either side of the spine. It is two fingers' distance from the spine between the fourth and fifth lumbar vertebrae.

Therapeutic Functions: Activating this point sends more Qi to the Large Intestine strengthening its energetic and physical functions.

Contra-Indications: None.

Guanyuanshu (Bladder Meridian 26) – 'Original Gate Delivery Point' – 關元俞

Guanyuanshu sits either side of the spine. It is two fingers' distance from the spine directly below the fifth lumbar vertebra.

Therapeutic Functions: Activating this point sends more Qi to the sexual organs which can help with sexual impotence and lack of libido. When this point is activated it is common to feel warmth spreading through the sexual organs which often leads to arousal.

Contra-Indications: None.

Suggested Points for Common Internal States

Below is a list of the internal conditions outlined in Chapter 8. For each internal imbalance there is a list of commonly selected points which can be activated in a single practice session to help redress this imbalance. This is just a very general overview of points which can be used. Each person will be unique and so the skill in this kind of practice is selecting a creative and useful combination of points to bring about positive change. I suggest that you use the lists here when you are starting out in your practice as they are safe and effective. Once you have begun to build up some confidence and experience you can begin to adjust the lists to suit your own unique needs.

Heart Yin Deficiency

- Lingdao (Heart 4)
- Shenmen (Heart 7) *unless there is also depression*
- Neiguan (Pericardium 6)
- Jiquan (Heart 1)

Heart Yang Deficiency

- Shenmen (Heart 7) *unless there is also depression*
- Neiguan (Pericardium 6)
- Fuliu (Kidney 7)
- Jiquan (Heart 1)

Heart Qi Deficiency

- Lingdao (Heart 4)
- Neiguan (Pericardium 6)
- Taiyuan (Lung 9)
- Mingmen (Governing Meridian 4)

Heart Blood Deficiency

- Lingdao (Heart 4)
- Shenmen (Heart 7) *unless there is also depression*
- Qihai (Conception Meridian 6)

Heart Fire

- Shaohai (Heart 3)
- Lingdao (Heart 4)
- Taixi (Kidney 3)

Heart Blood Stagnation

- Yongquan (Kidney 1)
- Jiquan (Heart 1)

It is unlikely that you would be using these practices in the dire situation of Heart Blood Stagnation but you never know what will happen in life!

Both of these points can be used in this situation. Yongquan is a last-ditch attempt at drawing in nourishing Earth energy.

Spleen Yang Deficiency

- Taibai (Spleen 3)
- Sanyinjiao (Spleen 6)
- Yinlingquan (Spleen 9)

Spleen Qi Deficiency

- Taibai (Spleen 3)
- Gongsun (Spleen 4)
- Sanyinjiao (Spleen 6)
- Tianshu (Stomach 25)

Cold in the Spleen

- Yinlingquan (Spleen 9)
- Gongsun (Spleen 4)
- Fenglong (Stomach 40)
- Mingmen (Governing Meridian 4)

Lung Yin Deficiency

- Chize (Lung 5)
- Taiyuan (Lung 9)
- Guanyuan (Conception Meridian 4)
- Zhaohai (Kidney 6)

Lung Qi Deficiency

- Taiyuan (Lung 9)
- Lieque (Lung 7)
- Zusanli (Stomach 36)
- Zhaohai (Kidney 6)

Wind Invasion of the Lungs

- Lieque (Lung 7)
- Shaoshang (Lung 11)
- Quchi (Large Intestine 11) *in the case of Wind Heat*

Phlegm in the Lungs

- Lieque (Lung 7)
- Chize (Lung 5)
- Shaoshang (Lung 11)

Kidney Yin Deficiency

- Taixi (Kidney 3)
- Guanyuan (Conception Meridian 4)
- Sanyinjiao (Spleen 6)

It is likely that you will also need to treat the back with points as described above.

Kidney Yang Deficiency

- Fuliu (Kidney 7)
- Guanyuan (Conception Meridian 4)
- Mingmen (Governing Meridian 4)

Kidney Qi Deficiency

- Taixi (Kidney 3)
- Qihai (Conception Meridian 6)
- Guanyuan (Conception Meridian 4)

Liver Yin Deficiency

- Taichong (Liver 3)
- Sanyinjiao (Spleen 6)
- Taixi (Kidney 3)

Liver Qi Deficiency

- Taichong (Liver 3)
- Sanyinjiao (Spleen 6)
- Zusanli (Stomach 36)

Liver Blood Deficiency

- Taichong (Liver 3)
- Sanyinjiao (Spleen 6)
- Guanyuan (Conception Meridian 4)
- Zusanli (Stomach 36)

Liver Blood Stasis

- Taichong (Liver 3)
- Hegu (Large Intestine 4) *coupled with Taichong this point promotes free movement*
- Qihai (Conception Meridian 6)
- Gongsun (Spleen 4)

Liver Yang Rising

- Xingjian (Liver 2)
- Taichong (Liver 3)
- Yongquan (Kidney 1)
- Huiyin (Conception Meridian 1) *to bring down the rising Qi*

Liver Fire

- Xingjian (Liver 2)
- Taichong (Liver 3)
- Quchi (Large Intestine 11)
- Taixi (Kidney 3) *to produce more water Qi*

Pericardium Qi Stagnation
- Daling (Pericardium 7)
- Zhongchong (Pericardium 9)

Pericardium Heat
- Laogong (Pericardium 8)
- Quze (Pericardium 3)
- Quchi (Large Intestine 11)

Heat in the Small Intestines
- Wangu (Small Intestine 4)
- Shaoze (Small Intestine 1)
- Quchi (Large Intestine 11)
- Tianshu (Stomach 25)

Small Intestine Qi Deficiency
- Wangu (Small Intestine 4)
- Houxi (Small Intestine 3)
- Taichong (Liver 3) *Yin Wood to nourish Yang Fire*

Damp Heat in the Stomach
- Chongyang (Stomach 42)
- Fenglong (Stomach 40)
- Quchi (Large Intestine 11)
- Tianshu (Stomach 25)

Stomach Fire
- Chongyang (Stomach 42)
- Tianshu (Stomach 25)
- Shousanli (Large Intestine 10)

Damp Heat in the Large Intestines

- Quchi (Large Intestine 11)
- Fenglong (Stomach 40)
- Hegu (Large Intestine 4)

Dry Large Intestines

- Yangxi (Large Intestine 5)
- Quchi (Large Intestine 11)
- Tianshu (Stomach 25)
- Hegu (Large Intestine 4)
- Taichong (Liver 3) *coupled with Hegu, this point promotes movement*

Damp Heat in the Bladder

- Quchi (Large Intestine 11)
- Yinlingquan (Spleen 9)
- Jingu (Bladder 64)

Deficient Bladder Qi

- Jingu (Bladder 64)
- Shenmai (Bladder 62)

Damp in the Gall Bladder

- Fenglong (Stomach 40)
- Yanglingquan (Gall Bladder 34)

Gall Bladder Qi Deficiency

- Yanglingquan (Gall Bladder 34)
- Shousanli (Large Intestine 10)
- Zusanli (Stomach 36)

Upper Jiao Weakness

- Yangchi (Triple Heater 4)
- Baihui (Governing Meridian 20)

Middle Jiao Weakness

- Yangchi (Triple Heater 4)
- Shanzhong (Conception Meridian 17)

Lower Jiao Weakness

- Yangchi (Triple Heater 4)
- Qihai (Conception Meridian 6)

Triple Heater Qi Deficiency

- Yangchi (Triple Heater 4)
- Mingmen (Governing Meridian 4)

Uterus Yang Deficiency

- Guanyuan (Conception Meridian 4)
- Mingmen (Governing Meridian 4)
- Fuliu (Kidney 7)

Uterus Yin Deficiency

- Guanyuan (Conception Meridian 4)
- Sanyinjiao (Spleen 6) *use this point directly after the new moon*

Cold in the Uterus

- Guanyuan (Conception Meridian 4)
- Qihai (Conception Meridian 6)
- Huiyin (Conception Meridian 1)

Marrow Deficiency

- Baihui (Governing Meridian 20)
- Taixi (Kidney 3)
- Fuliu (Kidney 7)

CHAPTER 12

CONCLUSION AND GOING FURTHER

This book has been an introduction to the process of exploring and understanding the human energy body using focused awareness and various internal exercises. As with any aspect of the Daoist arts which are recorded in written form, this book only scratches the surface. With time and practice it is possible to go much deeper into your own internal exploration and gain experiential understandings of your own. It is my hope that this book will help to spark the interest of those reading it and inspire internal practitioners to enrich their understanding of Daoism with personal exploration.

Qi Gong and Nei Gong sit somewhere between physical exercises and meditation. Daoist alchemical practices cross over with the exercises contained within this book and exploring the meridians, the Heavenly Streams, can serve as a bridge between Qi Gong and the deeper stages of attainment which can only be reached through Daoist sitting practices. It is also quite possible that the focused use of your mind combined with deep breathing will naturally begin to lead you towards stages that you had not originally aimed for. In my conclusion I would like briefly to introduce some of these internal attainments which can be had through practices such as those contained within the book. Indeed many of my students in the UK and abroad have experienced some of these stages. It often catches them by surprise as they expected alchemy to be the vehicle through which they reached these levels rather than internal exploration of the meridian system. Such is the unpredictable nature of Daoism, full of surprises!

The Breakdown of Reality

We have discussed at length throughout the previous chapters how Qi is simply a form of vibrational information which can be interpreted by the brain providing we are able to make contact with it. This information is read as heat, cold, pressure, pain and so forth, so that we are able to understand the nature of the energy we are reading. In the same way the brain translates the vibrational information of the Qi which surrounds us to make up the world we live in. All of our interactions with the physical world are dependent upon our brain's function of reading the Qi of the environment to give the impression of the outside world; this is the basis of many spiritual traditions across the world and a truth that people often experience when in altered states of consciousness. How does this happen? In order to understand this we need to look at the nature of how the brain reads the vibrational information of Jing, Qi and Shen.

The brain can only read information at one stage of energetic refinement above where it is primarily focused. For the majority of people the brain is interpreting information within the physical world, the realm of Jing. The physical matter of the world depends upon the Jing vibrational pattern of the objects with which we interact. One stage above Jing is Qi and so our brain is also interpreting the information of the energetic realm although it is often on a purely subconscious level. The readings of the energetic realm, Qi, will be subtle as our brain is primarily focused upon the physical world, Jing. Occasionally everybody will interpret the Qi around us and within the body but it is often put down to intuition. Obviously some people are naturally more inclined towards feeling the realm of Qi and these people are more able to interpret this information than the general population. These people are often called psychics and many of them work within the energy healing field. Figure 12.1 summarises the information usually interpreted by the brain.

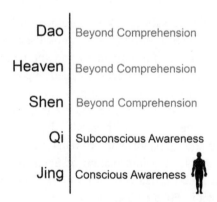

Dao	Beyond Comprehension
Heaven	Beyond Comprehension
Shen	Beyond Comprehension
Qi	Subconscious Awareness
Jing	Conscious Awareness

Figure 12.1: The Brain Focused Upon the Physical World

As you can see from Figure 12.1, the brain is not able to interpret the information contained within the realm of pure consciousness, Shen, and certainly does not connect with the realms of Heaven or pure emptiness, Dao. This is because Shen is two steps away from Jing while Heaven and Dao are three and four steps away from Jing.

When we are able to carry out the practices contained within this book we shift our brain's ability to interpret information. The focus of the brain shifts primarily to the energetic realm, Qi, once we are comfortably able to contact our meridian system. Jing is one step away from Qi and so we will still also be in contact with the physical world. Now Shen is also only one step away from where our brain is primarily focused and so we can begin to interpret information directly from the realm of pure consciousness. Figure 12.2 summarises the focus of the brain during internal practices such as those contained within this book.

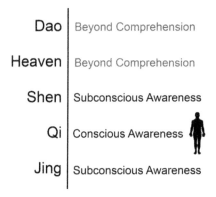

Figure 12.2: The Brain Focused Upon the Energetic World

Since we are now able to subtly pick up information from the realm of pure consciousness, Shen, it is likely that we will experience profound insights into the nature of our own mind and the nature of the world within which we live. These experiences depend upon us being able to remain in a focused internal state for long periods of time and many of the insights associated with those who practise meditation are the result of this contact with Shen. Those with minds who still fluctuate between contacting the Jing and Qi realms will not remain in a state long enough for the brain to interpret the information of Shen to any great degree. Much of this book is concerned with bringing the brain into the state of interpretation shown in Figure 12.2.

The 'breakdown of reality' is something often documented within the Eastern arts. It is associated with the realisation that the nature of physicality is essentially false. Not only is the physical world mostly empty space but its existence is also a very subjective matter. Once again this is a concept which must be directly experienced in order to understand it; it is not a concept which can easily be understood through intellectual study but nonetheless I will attempt to explain it through the language of

Daoism. When the brain refines its interpretation to an even higher level then it will contact the realm of Shen directly. This is generally a very natural progression which takes place mainly through meditative practices but it can also happen through the exercises contained within this book which is why I have included information on it here. Figure 12.3 shows the focus of the brain during the breakdown of reality.

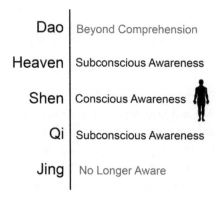

Dao	Beyond Comprehension
Heaven	Subconscious Awareness
Shen	Conscious Awareness
Qi	Subconscious Awareness
Jing	No Longer Aware

Figure 12.3: The Breakdown of Reality

In Figure 12.3 the brain is focused upon the realm of Shen. Qi is only one stage below Shen but Jing is now two stages of refinement away. This means that the brain is now no longer able to interpret the information contained within the Jing of the physical world. The result of this is that the physical world dissolves. There is no connection between the brain and Jing so there is no longer any physical body and no world for it to exist within. Instead we experience the nature of pure consciousness with a root in the energetic realm. The result is total expansion and interconnectedness of everything. Division is based within the physical realm of Jing while union is based within the realms of Qi and Shen. This is a deeply transformative stage which can serve to 'reset' many aspects of the mind and body leading to miraculous changes to our health and nature.

Many practitioners of the internal arts who reach this level of attainment make drastic changes to their lives after they have experienced the profound oneness of direct contact with Shen and the breakdown of reality. This stage is greatly seductive and the feeling once leaving this state is often one of disappointment. I remember the intense urge to get back to this state of mind after I first experienced it. Like a drug it took a hold of my mind for a long time leaving me frustrated when my practices did not enable me to dissolve the physical world. It was only when I finally gave in and resigned myself to never experiencing it again that I once again found my brain directly interpreting the vibrational information of Shen. It is a truth which runs through all of the spiritual arts that 'striving' leads to nothing but dead ends.

There is an old story which illustrates this fact:

> An old monk sat with his student on a mountain's edge looking out over the world below. The young apprentice asked of his master 'How long will it take me to attain enlightenment master?' The master looked at his student, pondered for a while and answered 'It will take you around ten years.' The apprentice looked somewhat deflated and then asked 'What if I practice really hard and dedicate 100 per cent of my effort towards this goal?' Laughing, the master replied 'At least twenty years.'

The realms of Heaven and Dao which sit at vibrational levels above Shen can be contacted at later stages in your internal practices. These require advanced alchemical teachings and a qualified master who can lead you towards the final goal of complete union with Dao. At this stage not only does the physical world cease to exist but also the realms of Qi and Shen. This is the complete dissolving of self which leads to a person merging with the original entity of Dao. These stages are currently beyond my own understanding or ability and so I cannot write about them with any kind of authority.

Inner Vision

An interesting experience to be had from the practice of internal exploration is using the ability known as 'inner vision'. Once again this seems to develop naturally from prolonged practice of the exercises outlined within this book. When I first started talking about this, many of my students were sceptical. Now quite a few of them have experienced it for themselves and so they have been forced to reject their scepticism.

When the brain is focused primarily on the realm of Qi it can begin to interpret the information contained within the meridians in different ways. At early stages the brain will read the vibrational information of Qi to give feelings of heat, cold and all of the other sensations outlined within this book. Each of these can obviously be used as an indicator of a different quality or movement of energy within the body or environment. At later stages the brain begins to decode the Qi in different ways and so will begin to give you visual information. The result of this is that you will begin to be able to see your own meridian system.

With your eyes closed you are shutting off any outside visual information and as the Yi contacts the meridians it brings up a clear image of the nature of the Qi which flows through you. With practice it is even possible to direct your Yi through the body and so travel through the meridian system 'looking' at the Qi which flows through your body. I remember being surprised by the complexity of the meridian system when I first saw it for myself. I imagined a series of pathways which could clearly be identified as individual meridians but instead I was confronted by a mass of silver, glittering streams which look like a tangled up pile of silver string. The chance of being able to pick out an individual meridian among the mass of the meridian system is very slim indeed. This mass of tangled energetic pathways continues throughout the whole body. I have heard of practitioners who are able to use this ability to see their own organs as well but unfortunately I am unable to do this so I cannot describe the experience in any way. My own inner vision is linked to the realm of Qi but I have no doubt whatsoever that the brain can decode the realm of internal Jing into visual information as well, giving an image of individual organs.

The Wuji of the Chong Mai

One last experience I should discuss is the nature of the Chong Mai as it can be experienced through the practices in this book. The central branch of the Chong Mai runs vertically through our body as shown in Figure 12.4.

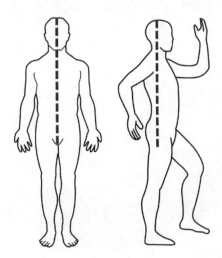

Figure 12.4: The Central Branch of the Chong Mai

The central branch of the Chong Mai is said to be the area of the energy body which contacts the realm of Wuji directly. It is from this vertical branch of spiritual information that everything grows outwards once the seed of consciousness has been planted within the spiritual realm. If we are able to send our Yi into the centre of the Chong Mai then we are able to experience the nature of Wuji which sits within the centre of our energy body. Generally this is accomplished through particular meditational practices within the Daoist tradition but I have included information on this experience here since it is also possible to stumble across the centre of the Chong Mai accidentally through the practices outlined in this book.

It is from the state of Wuji that the seed consciousness first appears; it is from here that the vibrational patterns of Shen, Qi and then finally Jing manifest. If we make contact with Wuji then we will experience our original state prior to the formation of our consciousness. This is a state of complete mental and emotional emptiness. Figure 12.5 shows the location of Wuji within the Chong Mai and the aspects of consciousness which are born from it.

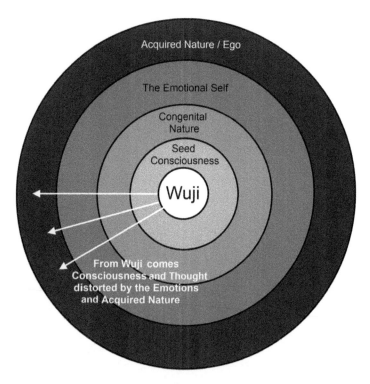

Figure 12.5: Wuji and the Consciousness

As you can see from the above diagram, from out of our consciousness come our emotions. These constantly fluctuating waves of information sit somewhere between the realms of Shen and Qi meaning that excessive disturbances here can begin to develop imbalances within both the mind and the energy body; over time these imbalances lead to physical sickness. If we think of emotional stability as being a centre point then every emotion we experience moves us away from this centre. This in itself is not a problem providing that once the emotion has passed we move back to this centre point. It is healthy and natural to have emotions but they can become detrimental to our health when we have an excess of one particular emotional state. Staying for long periods of time in this emotional state means that we never fully return to the central point of emotional stability which we are striving for within the Daoist internal arts. It is a sad fact that almost nobody ever experiences this central point of stability as we are bombarded by external factors which lead to emotional swings from the second we are conceived. We all have a tendency towards one or more emotional states and so one or more emotional energies which have a constant negative effect upon our health as discussed previously in this book.

If we are able to contact the realm of Wuji which sits at the centre of our Chong Mai we will experience this elusive state of emotional stability. For many people this is one of the most profound experiences they will ever have. To feel what it is like to have no strong emotional imbalance shows you what it feels like to contact your original state of being. This is the state of Wuji. It is in this state that you will first understand the reason for the way that you are. Great insights into your motives can be gained from this experience which for many people can also be very difficult. The truth as to why you do the things you do can be quite a slap in the face. From a personal perspective I was disappointed with myself to discover that many of the kind actions I did for other people were actually for myself; that which I thought I did solely for the good of others was actually to massage some deep wound left my an emotional imbalance within myself. Understanding this enabled me to move towards rebalancing this aspect of myself although it was a painful realisation to come to. While I am nowhere near keeping myself at this balanced point of emotional centeredness I am confident that the experiences of Wuji I have had through my practices have given me the knowledge to begin working in the right direction. This has been a very healing process for me and I hope that others will be able to benefit from this experience as well.

In Conclusion

While many of the practices in this book are fairly difficult, they are attainable by anybody who is willing to put in the correct amount of time and effort. They form part of the foundational skills for any of the internal arts and so should, in my personal opinion, become a regular practice for any serious follower of Daoism.

The search for a state of internal balance and good health is an important part of anybody's life. Those who do not take the time to look after their own health ultimately end up paying the price. In a time when many people seem to be happy to depend upon others to look after their failing health I hope that these practices will inspire and empower some people to take the responsibility for their health into their own hands. Having a way to contact your own body at an energetic level is a great boon for those who wish to remain healthy and content. It is only from here that we can easily move forward towards deeper levels of cultivation. The path towards spiritual elevation should be built upon a foundation of good health and energetic balance. This relies upon a smooth, healthy flow of Qi, a good level of exercise, a good diet, a healthy mind and harmonisation with the great powers of Heaven and Earth. While this may be a long road to follow it is a rewarding one and so I will end this book by reminding you of the most important part of any internal practice… Enjoy yourself.

GLOSSARY OF PINYIN TERMS

The following glossary of Pinyin terms contains Chinese terminology used throughout this book. Simplified Chinese characters have been included for reference purposes apart from where traditional Chinese characters are still commonly used as in the case of Chinese medical terminology.

Baihui 百會 (GV20) An acupuncture point situated on top of the head. Translated as meaning 'hundred meetings' due to it being the meeting place for the six Yang meridians. In classical Daoism it is also the point where numerous spirits converge.

Da Zhou Tian 大周天 'Large Heavenly cycle' also known as the large water wheel of Qi. This is the primary circulation of energy out of the body which can be achieved through consistent alchemy or Nei Gong training.

Dan Tien 丹田 Usually refers to the lowest of the three main 'elixir fields'. Its primary function is the conversion of Jing to Qi and moving the Qi throughout the meridian system.

Dao 道 The nameless and formless origin of the universe. Daoism is the study of this obscure concept and all internal arts are a way of experientially understanding the nature of Dao.

Dao De Jing 德道经 The 'virtue of following the way'. The classical text of Daoism written by the great sage Laozi. Also written as *Dao De Ching*.

De 德 The congenital manifestation of the transient emotions. De is born from deep within the true human consciousness which is usually buried beneath the various layers of the Ego.

Dui 兑 One of the eight Trigrams of Daoist Bagua theory. Its energetic manifestation is metaphorically likened to a lake although Dui does not directly mean lake.

Feng Shui 风水 'Wind and water'. This is the Daoist study of environmental energies and the influence of the macrocosm upon the human energy system and consciousness.

Gen 艮 One of the eight Trigrams of Daoist Bagua theory. Its energetic manifestation is likened to that of a mountain.

Gua 卦 'Trigram'. These are the eight sacred symbols which make up Daoist Bagua theory. They are a way to conceptualise the various vibrational frequencies of the energetic realm and how they interact.

Huiyin 會陰 (CO1) 'Meeting of Yin' is an acupuncture point located at the perineum. It is named after the fact that it is situated within the most Yin area of the human body.

Hun 魂 'Yang soul' – the ethereal soul which continues to exist after our death. It is usually housed within the liver.

Ji Ben Qi Gong 基本气功 'Fundamental energy exercises': the eight basic level exercises outlined within this book. The primary exercises taught within the Lotus Nei Gong School of internal arts which is based in the UK.

Jing 精 The lowest vibrational frequency of the three main energetic substances of man. Usually translated as meaning 'essence' and often misunderstood as being human sexual fluids.

Jing Gong 精功 'Essence exercises' – the technique of building up and refining our Jing.

Jing Luo 经络 The human meridian system which is made up of numerous energetic pathways which regulate the body and transport Qi to and from our organs and tissues.

Jue Yin 厥阴 The terminal Yin aspect of the six divisions.

Kan 坎 One of the eight Trigrams of Daoist Bagua theory which is usually likened to the energetic manifestation of water.

Kun 坤 One of the eight Trigrams of Daoist Bagua theory. Its energetic manifestation is usually likened to that of the planet.

Laogong 劳宫 (PC8) An acupuncture point situated in the centre of the palm. Its name means 'palace of toil' due to it being on the human hand which carries out a lot of physical work. Within Daoism they also know this point to be very important in venting heat from the heart and so it is rarely at rest. Very important point in Qi Gong practice as it regulates the internal temperature and also allows us to emit Qi in practices such as external Qi therapy.

Laozi 老子 The great sage. The original Daoist who wrote the *Dao De Ching*, supposedly leaving this text with a border watchman when he retreated into isolation in the western mountains of China.

Li 離 One of the eight Trigrams of Daoist Bagua theory. Its energetic manifestation is usually likened to fire.

Ming 命 Your predestined journey from life to death. Usually translated as meaning 'fate' but this really does not explain the true meaning of the term.

Mingmen 命门 (GV4) An acupuncture point in the lower back which is very important in Nei Gong practise. This point is referred to several times in this book and serious internal arts practitioners should work very hard to awaken the energy in this area of their meridian system.

Nei Gong 内功 The process of internal change and development which a person may go through if they practise the internal arts to a high level.

Po 魄 The 'Yin soul' which dies with the human body. Largely connected to our physical sense; the Po resides in the lungs.

Qi 氣 'Energy'. A term that is often difficult to translate into English. In Nei Gong theory it is an energetic vibration which transports information through the energy system.

Qi Gong 氣功 Usually gentle exercises which combine rhythmic movements with breathing exercises to shift Qi through the body. The term means 'energy exercises' although it is sometimes translated as meaning 'breathing exercises'.

Qihai 氣海 (CO6) An acupuncture point which sits in front of the lower Dan Tien. Its name in English means 'sea of Qi' as it is the point from where Qi is generated and where it flows from. Like water returning to the sea in rivers and streams, Qi returns to the lower Dan Tien when it circulates in the 'small water wheel of Qi'.

Qian 乾 One of the eight Trigrams of Daoist Bagua theory. Its energetic manifestation is usually likened to the movements of Heaven.

Ren 人 Within Daoism, Ren is 'humanity'. Humanity sits between Heaven and Earth and is a reflection of their fluctuations and movements. Ren is nourished by Earth and stimulated to development through Heaven.

Shao Yang 少阳 The lesser Yang aspect of the six divisions.

Shao Yin 少阴 The lesser Yin aspect of the six divisions.

Shen 神 The energy of consciousness. Vibrates at a frequency close to that of Heaven. It is manifested within the body as a bright white light.

Shen Gong 神功 This is the arcane skill of working with the substance of consciousness. Within Daoism it is said that a skilled Shen Gong practitioner can manipulate the very energy of the environment.

Sun 巽 One of the eight Trigrams of Daoist Bagua theory. Its energetic manifestation is usually likened to that of the wind.

Sung 松 This is the process of transferring habitual tension from the physical or consciousness body into the energetic realm where it can be dissolved.

Tai ji 太极 A Daoist concept of creation which can be translated as meaning the 'motive force of creation'.

Tai Yang 太阳 The greater Yang aspect of the six divisions.

Tai Yin 太阴 The greater Yin aspect of the six divisions.

Tian 天 'Heaven'. Not to be mistaken for the Christian concept of Heaven; this refers to the vibrational frequency of the macrocosm. Within the microcosm of the body Heaven is used metaphorically to refer to human consciousness.

Tui Na 推拿 A form of Chinese medical massage which means 'push and grab'.

Wu Xing 五行 The five elemental energies which are an important part of Daoist creation theory, psychology and medicine.

Wu Xing Qi Gong 五行气功 'Five Element energy exercises'. The five medical exercises taught within this book. They are an important part of the Lotus Nei Gong syllabus.

Wuji 无极 The Daoist concept of non-existence. The blank canvas upon which reality is projected and an important part of Daoist creation philosophy.

Xin-Yi 心意 'Heart-Mind'. This is the framework with which we attempt to understand the various aspects of human consciousness. Originally a Buddhist concept, it was absorbed into Daoist teachings.

Yang Ming 阳明 The shining Yang aspect of the six divisions.

Yang Qi 阳氣 Our internal Qi which moves out towards the surface of the body and the congenital meridians.

Yang Shen Fa 养身法 Literally 'life nourishing principles'. This is the Daoist practice of living healthily which should be studied alongside all internal arts.

Yi 意 'Intention' or 'awareness'. An important element of human consciousness to cultivate in Nei Gong training.

Yi Jing 易经 The *Classic of Change*. An ancient Daoist text which is based upon Bagua theory.

Yin Qi 阴氣 Our internal Qi which moves in to nourish the organs of the body.

Ying Qi 营氣 The nutritive energy which primarily flows through the body within the physical vehicle of the Blood.

Yongquan 涌泉 (KI1) An acupuncture point on the base of the foot which means 'bubbling spring'. This is the main point through which Earth energy is drawn into the body.

Zang Fu 脏腑 The collective name for the Yin and Yang organs of the body.

Zhen 震 One of the eight Trigrams of Daoist Bagua theory. Its energetic manifestation is often likened to thunder.

Zhi 志 An element of human consciousness which is directly linked to the state of our kidneys. The nearest translation in English is 'will-power'.

Ziran 自然 The Daoist philosophical concept of acting in harmony with nature and returning to an original state.

RECOMMENDED READING

Bertschinger, R. (2011) *The Secret of Everlasting Life: The First Translation of the Ancient Chinese Text of Immortality*. London: Singing Dragon.

Cleary, T. (1986) *The Taoist I Ching*. Boston, MA: Shambhala Publications Inc.

Cleary, T. (1996) *Opening the Dragon Gate*. Boston, MA: Tuttle Publishing.

Deadman, P. (2007) *A Manual of Acupuncture*. Hove: Journal of Chinese Medicine Publications.

Maciocia, G. (1989) *The Foundations of Chinese Medicine*. Edinburgh: Churchill Livingstone.

Maoshing, N. (1995) *The Yellow Emperors Classic of Medicine*. Boston, MA: Shambhala Publishing Inc.

Mitchell, D. (2011) *Daoist Nei Gong: The Philosophical Art of Change*. London: Singing Dragon.

Reid, D. (1993) *Guarding the Three Treasures*. Sydney: Simon and Schuster.

Reid, D. (1998) *A Complete Guide to Chi Gung*. Boston, MA: Shambhala Publications Inc.

Waley, A. (1999) *Laozi*. Hunan: Hunan People's Publishing House.

ABOUT THE AUTHOR

Damo Mitchell was born into a family of martial artists and so began his training at the age of four. This training has continued throughout his life and expanded to include the study of both internal and external martial arts, meditation and Chinese medicine as well as Nei Gong. His studies have taken him across the planet in search of authentic masters of the spiritual traditions and he spends his time studying, travelling and teaching.

Damo is the technical director of the Lotus Nei Gong School of Daoist Arts, which is based in the UK and Sweden, where he teaches through a combination of intensive courses and long-term retreats that range from two days to several months in length. For more information on Damo and his teachings please visit his website: www.lotusneigong.com.

INDEX